AF745654

Hernia Surgery

Edited by Selim Sözen and Hasan Erdem

Published in London, United Kingdom

Hernia Surgery
http://dx.doi.org/10.5772/intechopen.98030
Edited by Selim Sözen and Hasan Erdem

Contributors
Ioannis Triantafyllidis, Rodolfo J. Oviedo, Jeffrey Hodges, Joseph Nguyen-Lee, David Detz, Mary Oh, Anuj Shah, João Bombardelli, Atteeba Manzar, Alessandro Martinino, Wasim Dar, Uday Muddebihal, Uliargoli Vasudeva Rao, Somprakas Basu, Aakansha Giri Goswami, Farhanul Huda, Navin Kumar, Sudhir Kumar Singh, Charalampos Seretis, Chrysanthi Papageorgopoulou, Fotios Odisseas Efthymiou, Konstantinos Nikolakopoulos, Michinobu Ohno, Yasushi Fuchimoto, Akihiro Fujino, Toshihiko Watanabe, Yutaka Kanamori, Bruno Barbosa, Maria João Diogo, César Prudente, Carlos Casimiro, Giovambattista Caruso, Giuseppe Evola, Mariapia Gangemi, Salvatore Antonio Maria Benfatto, Luigi Conti, Filippo Banchini, Carmine Grassi, Gaetano Maria Cattaneo, Edoardo Baldini, Patrizio Capelli, Deborah Bonfili, Selim Sözen, Seyfi Emir, Hasan Erdem, Mehmet Gençtürk, Muhammed Said Dalkılıç, Abdullah Şişik

© The Editor(s) and the Author(s) 2022
The rights of the editor(s) and the author(s) have been asserted in accordance with the Copyright, Designs and Patents Act 1988. All rights to the book as a whole are reserved by INTECHOPEN LIMITED. The book as a whole (compilation) cannot be reproduced, distributed or used for commercial or non-commercial purposes without INTECHOPEN LIMITED's written permission. Enquiries concerning the use of the book should be directed to INTECHOPEN LIMITED rights and permissions department (permissions@intechopen.com).
Violations are liable to prosecution under the governing Copyright Law.

Individual chapters of this publication are distributed under the terms of the Creative Commons Attribution 3.0 Unported License which permits commercial use, distribution and reproduction of the individual chapters, provided the original author(s) and source publication are appropriately acknowledged. If so indicated, certain images may not be included under the Creative Commons license. In such cases users will need to obtain permission from the license holder to reproduce the material. More details and guidelines concerning content reuse and adaptation can be found at http://www.intechopen.com/copyright-policy.html.

Notice
Statements and opinions expressed in the chapters are these of the individual contributors and not necessarily those of the editors or publisher. No responsibility is accepted for the accuracy of information contained in the published chapters. The publisher assumes no responsibility for any damage or injury to persons or property arising out of the use of any materials, instructions, methods or ideas contained in the book.

First published in London, United Kingdom, 2022 by IntechOpen
IntechOpen is the global imprint of INTECHOPEN LIMITED, registered in England and Wales, registration number: 11086078, 5 Princes Gate Court, London, SW7 2QJ, United Kingdom

British Library Cataloguing-in-Publication Data
A catalogue record for this book is available from the British Library

Additional hard and PDF copies can be obtained from orders@intechopen.com

Hernia Surgery
Edited by Selim Sözen and Hasan Erdem
p. cm.
Print ISBN 978-1-80355-519-5
Online ISBN 978-1-80355-520-1
eBook (PDF) ISBN 978-1-80355-521-8

We are IntechOpen,
the world's leading publisher of
Open Access books
Built by scientists, for scientists

5,800+
Open access books available

143,000+
International authors and editors

180M+
Downloads

156
Countries delivered to

Our authors are among the
Top 1%
most cited scientists

12.2%
Contributors from top 500 universities

WEB OF SCIENCE™

Selection of our books indexed in the Book Citation Index
in Web of Science™ Core Collection (BKCI)

Interested in publishing with us?
Contact book.department@intechopen.com

Numbers displayed above are based on latest data collected.
For more information visit www.intechopen.com

For EU product safety concerns:
IN TECH d.o.o., Prolaz Marije Krucifikse Kozulić 3, 51000 Rijeka, Croatia,
info@intechopen.com or visit our website at intechopen.com.

Meet the editors

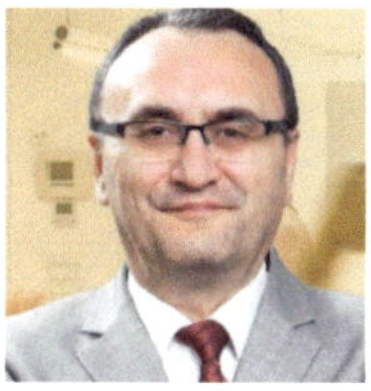

Dr. Selim Sözen is an expert in general surgery who received his medical degree from Ondokuz Mayıs University, Turkey, in 1998. From 1999 to 2004, he was an assistant doctor at Ankara Atatürk Education and Research Hospital, Turkey. From 2004 to 2013, he worked as a specialist at different government hospitals in Turkey. He joined the Department of General Surgery, Medicine Faculty, Namık Kemal University, Turkey, as an associate professor in 2013. He completed liver transplantation surgery at İnönü University, Turkey, in 2014–2015. Since 2016, Dr. Sözen has run his own surgery clinic in İstanbul, Turkey. He is a member of the Turkish Surgical Association and a review board member for several journals. He has published 109 articles in scientific journals and presented 64 poster papers at scientific congresses. His research interests include general, gastrointestinal, emergency, and trauma surgery, bacterial translocation, liver disease, and hernia surgery.

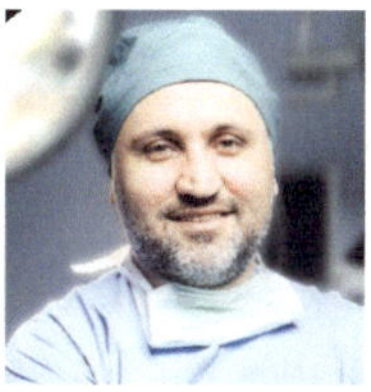

Dr. Hasan Erdem received his medical education between 1996 and 2002 at the Medical School of Istanbul University. In 2008, he completed his specialization in General Surgery at the Bezmialem Vakıf Gureba Teaching Hospital, Istanbul. Dr.Erdem was assigned to a state hospital where he performed his obligatory residency between 2009 and 2011. Upon completing his mandatory service, he worked as Chief Assistant in General Surgery at the Training and Research Hospital of Adana where he continued his studies in advanced laparoscopic and robotic surgery. In 2016, he established his private clinic in which he currently works. Dr. Erdem was granted the title Associate Professor of Obesity Surgery and Metabolic in 2018.

Contents

Preface

This book is a collection of review papers on hernia surgery. In addition to sharing their knowledge, the authors provide their personal clinical experience, making this book a useful resource for scientists and physicians practicing in the field of hernia surgery. Chapter 1, "Introductory Chapter: Abdominal Wall Hernias and Prosthetic Material" by Dr. Selim Sözen et al., examines the causes of hernia as well as discusses prosthetic material used in hernia repair such as synthetic, inorganic mesh patches. Chapter 2, "Anatomical and Surgical Principles of Ventral Hernia Repairs" by Dr. Charalampos Seretis et al., discusses anatomical and surgical principles of ventral hernia repairs. Chapter 3, "Totally Extraperitoneal Approach (TEP) for Inguinal Hernia Repair" by Dr. Ioannis Triantafyllidis, discusses laparoendoscopic inguinal hernia repair as the procedure of choice for the management of most primary recurrent inguinal hernias. Chapter 4, "Spigelian Hernia" by Dr. Bruno Barbosa et al., focuses on the intraperitoneal onlay mesh (IPO) approach. This procedure is a quick and technically less demanding approach that requires a shorter learning curve compared to others. IPOM does not require a peritoneal flap and surgeons are more familiar with the intra-abdominal anatomy. Chapter 5, "Spigelian Hernia: Clinical Features and Management" by Dr. Somprakas Basu et al., presents the differential diagnosis of spigelian hernia. Depending on its location, a spigelian hernia may mimic intra-abdominal pathologies, which can present with pain such as acute appendicitis, twisted ovarian cyst, tubo-ovarian pathologies, mesenteric lymphadenitis, biliary colic, peptic ulcer pain, pancreatic pain, or mesenteric ischemia. Chapter 6, "Laparoscopic Findings of Rare Pediatric Inguinal Hernias" by Dr. Michinobu Ohno et al., focuses on the laparoscopic percutaneous extraperitoneal closure (LPEC) procedure. It presents the laparoscopic findings of rare pediatric inguinal hernias. The advantages of the laparoscopic technique in pediatric hernias include accurate diagnosis, minimal pain, and cosmesis. Although laparoscopic repair of femoral hernia is established in adults, most pediatric surgeons choose the open approach. Chapter 7, "Laparoscopic TAPP Inguinal Hernia Repair" by Dr. Giovambattista Caruso et al., explores the transabdominal preperitoneal (TAPP) procedure, which is associated with immediate postoperative comfort, less chronic pain and numbness, less mesh infection, and a faster return to usual activities. Another advantage of the laparoscopic technique is the possibility of diagnosing and treating occult hernia during the same operation. The disadvantages of laparoscopic procedures are a longer learning curve with a greater risk of complications during the first 30–50 procedures and higher direct costs (general anesthesia, laparoscopic equipment, staples). Chapter 8, "Management of Obturator Hernia" by Dr. Luigi Conti et al., discusses obturator hernia, which is a rare entity. Its diagnosis is often unclear and should be included in the differential diagnosis of intestinal obstruction of unknown origin. Chapter 9, "Hybrid: Evolving Techniques in Laparoscopic Ventral Hernia Mesh Repair" by Dr. Wasim Dar et al., discusses techniques of ventral hernia repair. Laparoscopic ventral hernia mesh repair is the procedure of choice for most uncomplicated ventral hernias with smaller defects. For complicated, large, and multiple defects, the laparoscopic approach presents a big challenge and hence an open approach is used. A combination of laparoscopic and open techniques with minimal access avoids dissection of large subcutaneous flaps, early post-operative recovery, and comparable results. Chapter 10, "Robotic Complex Abdominal Wall Reconstruction: The Evolution of Component Separation" by Dr. Rodolfo J. Oviedo et al., encourages readers to enter the realm of robotic abdominal wall reconstruction Finally, Chapter 11, "Laparoscopic Hiatal Hernia Repair during in-Sleeve Gastrectomy" by Dr. Selim Sözen et al., discusses the limits and significance of the surgical management of hiatal hernia repair.

I thank the authors for their professional dedication and outstanding work in summarizing their clinical and research practices.

Selim Sözen
Associate Professor of General Surgery,
Sözen Surgery Clinic,
İstanbul, Turkey

Hasan Erdem
Associate Professor of General Surgery,
HE Obesity Clinic,
İstanbul, Turkey

Section 1

Introduction

Chapter 1

Introductory Chapter: Abdominal Wall Hernias and Prosthetic Material

Hasan Erdem, Seyfi Emir and Selim Sözen

1. Introduction

It is the displacement and protrusion of the intra-abdominal structure and organs from weak places on the abdominal wall. While there are many varieties, it most often occurs in the inguinal. Umbilical hernias follow. Due to the presence of intestine in the hernia sac, it is important because intestinal obstructions (knotting), fluid-electrolyte incompatibility and death are seen.

Hernias that occur in areas of abdominal surgery called inguinal, umbilical and incisional hernia are anterior abdominal wall hernias. Hiatal hernias, which are called as gastrocoele and cause reflux, are hernias at the junction of the stomach and esophagus.

It is observed in both sexes, but more in men.

As the causes of hernia; Sudden, severe increase in intra-abdominal pressure, infections with lung problems due to smoking, and in cases where chronic intra-abdominal pressure increases by coughing continuously, the anterior abdominal wall weakens and coughing time is prolonged

- Those with chronic obstructive pulmonary disease (COPD)
- In cases of increased intra-abdominal pressure in pregnant women
- In obese people (especially in people who have the weak anterior abdominal wall)
- In kidney patients who are dialyzed their peritoneal
- Abdominal wall hernia may develop in those with collagen vascular disease.

Anterior abdominal wall hernias; consist of a wide range of hernias including incision site, umbilical, epigastric and suprapubic hernias. Morbid obesity, accompanying diseases, immunosuppression and prostate diseases accompanied by urination disorders are known important factors in the formation of incisional hernias (IH). Although the first 5 years after surgery is the most critical time for the development of IHs, it can also develop later on [1]. After minimal invasive treatments commonly come into use, shorter hospital stays, reductions in wound site infections and recurrence rates have led to the increasing frequency of use of these methods [2–4]. A more comfortable view is provided by the magnification effect of the telescope in addition to the advantages such as laying the graft by seeing the minimal tissue trauma, graft and surrounding healthy tissue in detail in laparoscopic surgery, but experience is required for successful results together with these advantages. In a meta-analysis performed by Castro et al., it was found that laparoscopy reduced the postoperative hospital stay and the infection rate in the perioperative period, but increased the operative time, enterotomy, and postoperative pain [5]. Similarly, it was found that the duration of hospital stay, recurrence, complication and infection rates were lower in the laparoscopic group, but that the operation time was also shorter in the laparoscopic group in the study of Itani et al. [6].

Abdominal wall hernias (inguinal, femoral, umbilical, epigastric and incisional) require emergency surgery with a frequency of 5–13% due to incarceration. Following emergency surgery in incarcerated hernias, the risk of morbidity is still high despite advances in anesthesia, antisepsis, antibiotherapy, and fluid therapy [7, 8]. They reported 2% mortality in elective hernia operations, while this rate was 16% in emergency hernia operations in the research done by Williams and Hale [9]. There are many similar studies in the literature [10, 11].

Spigelian hernia is rarely seen and is also known as lateral ventral hernia. Spigelian hernia is the herniation of the peritoneal sac containing preperitoneal fat, peritoneal sac or rarely visceral from the Spigelian region. The Spigelian region is bounded laterally by the muscular fibers of the internal oblique and medially by the lateral edge of the anterior lamina of the rectus sheath. Spigelian hernia may be congenital or acquired. Although congenital Spigel hernia has been reported, it is mostly considered an acquired hernia. It constitutes 1–2% of all abdominal wall hernias. Incidence of incarceration and strangulation of Spigelian hernia is high [12–14]. Spigelian hernias are mostly observed in women. It was reported that it was found in women with a rate of 88% in some series [15]. The incidence probability of incarceration and strangulation is high because the neck of the hernia sac is narrow [16]. The need for emergency operation increases up to 20% [17]. Spigelian hernia should be treated surgically because of its high complications [18–20]. The closure can be done through the primary suture, patch or laparoscope [21].

Obturator hernia comprises for only 0.05–1.4% of all hernias [22]. Women are 6 to 9 times more at risk than men because of the wider pelvis. Conditions that increase intra-abdominal pressure such as advanced age, weight loss, constipation and chronic lung disease or ascites are other risk factors. Diagnosis of obturator hernia is usually difficult. Physical examination, ultrasonography, CT scan, laparoscopy, and laparotomy are useful. Early diagnosis of obturator hernia prevents complications such as strangulation and perforation, and thereby reduces mortality and morbidity. In respect to treatment of obsturator hernia, abdominal, retropubic, obturator, and inguinal surgical approaches have been used in case of non-emergency. However, in case of emergency, the abdominal approach should be preferred to research complications such as strangulation or perforation. The hernia sac should be attached by turning upside down after the sac shrinks. The stump should be repaired with mesh, Teflon, fascial flap, or primary sutures. It may also be covered by a segment of the omentum. For obturator hernia, laparoscopic approaches have also been described in the last 20 years [23, 24].

Supravesical hernias develop at the supravesical fossa between the remnants of the urachus and the left or right umbilical artery. They are often the cause of intestinal obstruction. The supravesical fossa is the abdominal wall area between the remnants of the urachus (median umbilical ligament) and the left or right umbilical artery (medial umbilical ligament) [25, 26]. The remnant of the urachus divides into the right and left fossa. There are two variants of supravesical hernias: an external form caused by the laxity of the vesical preperitoneal tissue, and an internal one with a growing hernia sac from back to front and above the bladder in a sagittal paramedian direction [25, 27]. External supravesical hernia often occurs as a direct inguinal hernia.

Congenital anomalies of the diaphragm are the result of fusion defects of the diaphragm, or these are due to intestinal developmental disorders accompanied with diaphragmatic closure problems. Congenital Diaphragmatic Hernias (CDH) are classified as Bochdalek (posterior-lateral), Morgagni (anterior-retrosternal) and septum transversum defects. Bochdalek Hernia is a congenital diaphragmatic anomaly that occurs in one in 2000–12,500 live births [28]. Surgical treatment of CDH can be performed by laparotomy, thoracotomy, laparoscopy, thoracoscopy and/or a combination of these procedures. Diaphragm defects can be closed with or without a prosthesis. Generally, closure of these defects with primary sutures is usually impossible due to the size of the defect. Various grafts can be used in this kind of hernias. Yet, although polyprolene mesh support provides for tissue growth, it is a theoretically accepted risk for this mesh to erode the gastrointestinal organs. By virtue of less adhesion formation in polytetrafluoroethylene and other dual prostheses, these grafts are more preferred [29].

After coming into use of laparoscopic techniques in general surgery in the 1990s, it has been reported that the first inguinal hernia repair was performed by method of minimal invasive in 1992 [30]. Transabdominally (TAPP) and Total extraperitoneal (TEP) methods are two important laparoscopic repair methods of inguinal hernia. The main difference between the TAPP and TEP method is the access to the preperitoneal space. TEP method is more suitable for patients with intra-abdominal adhesions due to not entering the abdomen [31]. Because of the advantage of abdominal exploration, the TAPP method may be more suitable for laparoscopic repair of strangulated hernias [31]. The learning curve in the TAPP method is shorter than the TEP method [32]. While using the TEP method, in case of technical problems, it may be turned the TAPP method instead of the open method. Success in inguinal hernia repair is associated with long-term recurrence rates, and these rates have been reported in the range of 1–2% for the TEP method and 0–3% for the TAPP method [33, 34]. It is considered that the TEP is more appropriate in patients with intra-abdominal adhesions, and the TAPP method in cases where extensive exploration.

2. Prosthetic material

As well as the surgery, developed by Italian surgeon Eduardo Bassini in the nineteenth century and called own name, opened an era in hernia surgery, the especially long-term results of hernia repairs were not at an acceptable level until the 1990s, when patch repair started to become popular. Likewise in such old methods, the individual's own tissues were brought closer to each other with suture and a serious distention was formed in the operation area. This distention caused severe pain and discomfort in the early postoperative period, delayed return to normal activities and work, and recurrence of the disease in the long term. In hernia surgeries, the fact that the results of traditional repairs performed by suturing the tissues each other are not sufficient, in other words, the high recurrence rate of hernia has led surgeons to consider different methods over time. Today, the patches used in hernia repairs (*mesh*) are mostly synthetic materials. In a word, it is a kind of prosthesis made of inorganic materials (*prosthetic material*).

3. Ideal patch

A patch to be placed on the human body for hernia surgeries should have certain features:

- The patch should be able to be produced in the desired structure, shape and size.
- It should be made from a non-carcinogenic substance that is to say not cause cancer.
- It should not cause allergic and hypersensitivity reactions.
- It should be able to integrate into human tissue, but not cause excessive inflammation and foreign reaction.
- It should have the strength to withstand the mechanical stress due to intra-abdominal pressure and abdominal wall movements.
- It should be chemically inert, that is to say, it should not react with tissue fluids.
- It should be able to sterilize.

Standard polypropylene (plastic) patch still takes the largest share among synthetic patches used in hernia surgeries. The standard polypropylene patch is a "small pore and high weight" prosthetic material. Compound patches are made partly from polypropylene and partly from materials that are absorbed and lost by body fluids over time. The solute may be polyglycolic acid or polyglecapron. Compound patches have sufficient resistance in all cases and can be used safely in the treatment of abdominal wall hernias. These patches find use especially in surgical incision hernias that require large patches.

In patches of dual mesh/composite mesh, the main material is usually polypropylene or sometimes polyester. The interior surface of the patch that will come into touch with the intestines is covered with some non-adhesive materials in order to prevent these risks. Because this process requires special technology, the cost of this kind of patches is high. Such expensive patches must use in the laparoscopic repair of ventral hernias (umbilical, epigastric, incisional, Spigelian). In addition, these patches are also needed for the open repair of hernias in which a part of the abdominal wall is lost or the tissues are impossible being closed up each other.

Biological patches are produced from donor tissue with advanced technology in a laboratory environment. Living tissues used for this purpose today are human, pig and bovine skin, pig small intestine submucosa tissue, bovine and horse pericardium (heart membrane). The grafts (patches) used in this approach, which can be called a kind of graft, are designed to form a suitable basis for later collagen production and storage, as well as they are rich in collagen material that will provide strength.

Author details

Hasan Erdem[1], Seyfi Emir[2] and Selim Sözen[3]*

1 Department of General Surgery, Istanbul Obesity Surgery (IOC), Kurtköy Ersoy Hospital, Istanbul, Turkey

2 Department of General Surgery, Reyap Çorlu Hospital, Tekirdağ, Turkey

3 Department of General Surgery, Sözen Surgery Clinic, Istanbul, Turkey

*Address all correspondence to: selimsozen63@yahoo.com

IntechOpen

© 2022 The Author(s). Licensee IntechOpen. This chapter is distributed under the terms of the Creative Commons Attribution License (http://creativecommons.org/licenses/by/3.0), which permits unrestricted use, distribution, and reproduction in any medium, provided the original work is properly cited.

References

[1] Barbaros U, Asoglu O, Seven R, Erbil Y, Dinccag A, Deveci U, et al. The comparison of laparoscopic and open ventral hernia repairs: A prospective randomized study. Hernia. 2007;**11**(1):51-56

[2] Othman H, Methwally YH, Bakr IS, Amer YA, Gaber MB, Egohary SA. Comparative study between laparoscopic and open repair of paraumbilical hernia. Journal of the Egyptian Society of Parasitology. 2012;**42**:175-182

[3] Hussain D, Sarfraz SL, Kasmani JS, Baliga KS, Ibrahim M, Syed HS, et al. Laparoscopic repair of ventral hernia. Journal of the College of Physicians and Surgeons–Pakistan. 2012;**22**:683-685

[4] Heniford BT, Park A, Ramshaw BJ. Laparoscopic repair of ventral hernias. A nine year experience with 850 consecutive hernias. Annals of Surgery. 2003;**238**:391-400

[5] Castro PMV, Rabelato JT, Monteiro GGR, Guerra GCD, Mazzurana M, et al. Laparoscopy versus laparotomy in the repair of ventral hernias: Systematic review and meta-analysis. Arquivos de Gastroenterologia. 2014;**51**(3):205-211

[6] Itani KM, Neumayer L, Reda D, Kim L, Anthony T. Repair of ventral incisional hernia: The design of a randomized trial to compare open and laparoscopic surgical techniques. American Journal of Surgery. 2004; **188**(6S):22-29

[7] Kulah B, Kulacoglu IH, Oruc MT, Duzgun AP, Moran M, Ozmen MM, et al. Presentation and outcome of incarcerated external hernias in adults. American Journal of Surgery. 2001;**181**:101-104

[8] Derici H, Unalp HR, Bozdag AD, Nazli O, Tansug T, Kamer E. Factors affecting morbidity and mortality in incarcerated abdominal wall hernias. Hernia. 2007;**11**:341-346

[9] Williams JS, Hale HW. The advisability of inguinal herniorrhaphy in the elderly. Surgery, Gynecology & Obstetrics. 1966;**122**:100-104

[10] Tingwald GR, Cooperman M. Inguinal and femoral hernia repair in geriatric patients. Surgery, Gynecology and Obstetrics. 1982;**154**:704-706

[11] Nehme AE. Groin hernias in elderly patients. Management and prognosis. American Journal of Surgery. 1983;**146**:257-260

[12] Skandalakis PN, Zoras O, Skandalakis JE, Mirilas P. Spigelian hernia: Surgical anatomy, embryology, and technique of repair. The American Surgeon. 2006;**72**(1):42-48

[13] Rauth T, Holzman M, Tarpley J. Spigelian, lumbar and obturator herniation. In: Cameron JL, editor. Current Surgical Therapy. 9th ed. Philadelphia: Elsevier Mosby; 2008. pp. 576-581

[14] Skandalakis LJ, Gadacz TR, Mansberger AR. Modern Hernia Repair. 1st ed. New York: Parthenon Publishing Com; 2002

[15] Malazgirt Z, Topgul K, Sokmen S, Ersin S, Turkcapar AG, Gok H, et al. Spigelian hernias: A prospective analysis of baseline parameters and surgical outcome of 34 consecutive patients. Hernia. 2006;**10**(4):326-330

[16] Moreno-Egea A, Flores B, Girela E, Martín JG, Aguayo JL, Canteras M.

Spigelian hernia: Bibliographical study and presentation of a series of 28 patients. Hernia. 2002;**6**(4):167-170

[17] Hermosa R, Prats A, Liendo M. Spigelian hernia. Personal experience and review of the literature. Revista Española de Enfermedades Digestivas. 2010;**102**(10):583-586

[18] Spangen L. Spigelian hernia. In: Nyhus LM, Condon RE, editors. Nyhus and Condon's Hernia. 4th ed. Philadelphia: Lippincott; 1995. pp. 381-392

[19] Nursal TZ, Kologlu M, Aran O. Spigelian hernia presenting as an incarcerated incisional hernia. Hernia. 1997;**1**(3):149-150

[20] Rogers FB, Camp PC. A strangulated Spigelian hernia mimicking diverticulitis. Hernia. 2001;**5**(1):51-52

[21] Larson DW, Farley DR. Spigelian hernias: Repair and outcome for 81 patients. World Journal of Surgery. 2002;**26**(10):1277-1281

[22] Chang SS, Shan YS, Lin YJ, Tai YS, Lin PW. A review of obturator hernia and a proposed algorithm for its diagnosis and treatment. World Journal of Surgery. 2005;**29**:450-454

[23] Bryant TL, Umstot RK Jr. Laparoscopic repair of an incarcerated obturator hernia. Surgical Endoscopy. 1996;**10**:437-438

[24] Yokoyama T, Kobayashi A, Kikuchi T, Hayashi K, Miyagawa S. Transabdominal preperitoneal repair for obturator hernia. World Journal of Surgery. 2011;**35**:2323-2327

[25] Jan YT, Jeng KS, Liu YP, Yang FS. Internal supravesical hernia. American Journal of Surgery. 2008;**196**:27-28

[26] Gwynedd Y. Supravesicul hernia: Rare cause of intestinal obstruction. International Journal of Surgery. 2008;**6**:471-472

[27] Saravanan B, Paramu MKA, Ranganathan E. Supravesical hernia: A rare cause of intestinal obstruction. International Journal of Surgery. 2008;**6**:471-472

[28] Goh BK, Teo MC, Chng SP, Soo KC. Right-sided Bochdalek's hernia in an adult. American Journal of Surgery. 2007;**194**:390-391

[29] Toydemir T, Akıncı H, Tekinel M, et al. Laparoscopic repair of an incarcerated bochdalek hernia in an elderly man. Clinics (São Paulo, Brazil). 2012;**67**:199-201

[30] Arregui ME, Davis CJ, Yucel O, Nagan RF. Laparoscopic mesh repair of inguinal hernia using a preperitoneal approach: A preliminary report. Surgical Laparoscopy Endoscopy & Percutaneous Techniques. 1992;**2**(1):53-58

[31] Bansal VK, Krishna A, Ghosh N, Bittner R, Misra MC. Comparison TAPP vs TEP: Which technique is better? In: Laparo-endoscopic Hernia Surgery. Berlin: Springer; 2018. pp. 151-170

[32] Bansal VK, Krishna A, Ghosh N, Bittner R, Misra MC. TAPP versus TEP– welche Technik ist besser? In: Laparo-Endoskopische Hernienchirurg. Berlin: Springer; 2018. pp. 159-180

[33] Lau H, Patil N, Yuen W, Lee F. Prevalence and severity of chronic groin pain after endoscopic totally extraperitoneal inguinal hernioplasty. Surgical Endoscopy. 2003;**17**(10):1620-1623

[34] Weiser H, Klinge B. Endoscopic hernia repair-experiences and characteristic features. Viszeralchirurgie. 2000;**35**(5):316-320

Section 2

Advances in Hernia Surgery

Chapter 2

Anatomical and Surgical Principles of Ventral Hernia Repairs

Chrysanthi Papageorgopoulou, Konstantinos Nikolakopoulos, Fotios Efthymiou and Charalampos Seretis

Abstract

Hernias comprise a growing problem in surgical science. The most recent classification scheme for hernias emphasizes on the size of defect as well as on whether it is an incisional hernia. The latter group includes complex hernias, namely hernias that can not be managed with simple surgical techniques. This can be accomplished with retromuscular repairs or the more complex anterior and posterior component separation techniques. An anatomic repair is usually reinforced with interposition of mesh. Newest techniques, such as the use of botulinum toxin to induce temporary paralysis of the lateral abdominal wall musculature, referred to as chemical component separation, now present new tools in the restoration of anatomy-based repairs. The chapter entitled "Anatomical and surgical principles of ventral hernia repairs" aims to describe the anatomical and surgical principles of current practice regarding the repair of ventral -primary and incisional-hernias.

Keywords: hernia, ventral, surgery, anatomy

1. Introduction

Ventral hernias constitute a significant percentage of abdominal wall hernias, making the topic of relevant surgical anatomy and operative principles a fundamental one for the general surgeons, as well as urologists, gynecologists and vascular surgeons who perform operations within the peritoneal cavity. Historically, their management can be as simple as placement of a few interrupted sutures to close the hernia defect, but can also be as demanding as a complex abdominal wall reconstruction for patients with loss of domain. Without a doubt, knowledge of the basic surgical anatomy principles and up-to-date operative techniques is mandatory for the avoidance of perioperative complications and reduction of future hernia recurrences. In this chapter, we aim to address these theoretical and practical issues, aiming to facilitate the formation of a structured individualized approach for the operating surgeons.

2. Principles of surgical anatomy of the anterior abdominal wall

The anterior abdominal wall is an anatomically complex structure, comprising of skin, subcuticular adipose tissue, myofascial complexes and parietal peritoneum. Its central component is formed by the muscle fibers of the rectus abdominis, which are encased within an aponeurotic sheath and extend from the costal margins to the pubis [1, 2]. The anterior and posterior layers of these sheaths fuse in the midline, forming the linea alba [3]. The lateral border of the recti muscles have a convex shape which forms the semilunar line [4]. Lateral to the rectus sheath, three distinct muscles are identified: the external oblique, internal oblique and transversus abdominis muscles [5]. The external oblique muscle lies most superficially of the three and runs in an inferior and medial direction. Immediately deep to that, the internal oblique muscle is encountered coursing in a crossing direction to the external oblique muscle fibers. Finally, the deepest-lying muscle is the transversus abdominis, which travels, in accordance to its name, in a transverse direction. Of particular importance to the surgical repair of the ventral hernias are the aponeuroses which invest the above-mentioned anterior abdominal wall muscles muscles and form the fascial sheath of the recti muscles, apart from investing their native muscle. Having as a landmark the arcuate line (or semicircular line of Douglas), which forms the axis between the right and left anterior superior iliac spines, the anterior rectus sheath is formed mainly by the external oblique aponeurosis and the external layer of the internal oblique aponeurosis, while he posterior rectus sheath is formed by the internal layer of the internal oblique aponeurosis, the transversus abdominis aponeurosis and the transversalis fascia. Inferiorly to the level of the arcuate line, the anterior rectus sheath is formed by layers of the aponeurosis of the external oblique, internal oblique and transverses abdominis muscles, while the posterior rectus sheath is absent, with transversalis fascia being the only pre-peritoneal fascial component of the recti complex [6]. Regarding its blood supply, the vast majority of inflow comes from the inferior and superior epigastric arteries, as well as complexes of the subcostal and lumbar arteries; venous outflow follows the main arterial branches [7, 8]. Finally, innervation is originating from the thoracic and lumbar spine, and more specifically between the levels of T4-L1 spinal nerves [9]. From a technical perspective, perforating branches encountered during the dissection of the subcuticular layer flaps are critical for the viability of the anterior abdominal wall skin and should be preserved as possible; the same accounts for the neurovascular bundles which are encountered during dissection along the retrorectus space, as they are absolutely vital for the perfusion and functionality of the anterior abdominal wall [10, 11].

3. Types of ventral hernias

With the term "ventral hernia" we tend to describe the epigastric hernias, umbilical/paraumbilical hernias, as well as the anterior abdominal wall incisional hernias [12]. Epigastric hernia any primary hernia located in the epigastric region of the anterior abdominal wall, topographically located anywhere on the axis of linea alba between the xiphoid process and 1–2 cm superiorly to the umbilical ring. They represent a true anatomical defect between the avascular fibers of the linea alba and usually contain pre-peritoneal adipose tissue, greater omentum, parts of the small or large bowel [13]. Very infrequntly the stomach or even the solid organs of the upper abdomen, have been reported to protrude through large epigastric hernia defects, however these reports are rather scarce in the literature [14]. It has to be noted, that in many individuals, there is a laxity of the linea alba and the anterior abdominal wall myofascial complexes, which clinically can manifestate as a "bulge" during Valsalva's maneuver between the recti muscles in the epigastric region and not surpisingly can be mistaken as a ventral hernia. This condition, in which only laxity of the linea alba exists without the presence of a defined, true anatomical defect exists, is called deverication of recti and its operative managment is completely different of a typical ventral hernia [15]. Therefore, the operating surgeon should have a low threshold for assesing these patients with a further imaging modality (ie ultasound, compute tomography or dynamic magnetic resonance scans) to confidently differentiate between the two conditions.

Umbilical/paraumbilical hernias, as the onomatology implies, are the hernias whose defects arise through or adjacent to the umbilical ring, and can be congential or develop later in life. Of note, the vast majority of the umbilical hernia defects that can be seen in infancy, will self-obliterate by the 5th year of age in more than three quarters of the patients [16]. With respect to those hernias arising during adult life, any factor which can increase the intra-abdominal pressure (obesity, ascites, chronic cough, pregnancy, chronic straining due to constipation) or weaken the strength of the anterior abdominal wall (connective tissue diseases, smoking, auto-immune disorders), could be implicated in their pathogenesis [17].

Incisional hernias occur at the sites of previous sites of surgical incisions and hence commonly are encountered in the midline (laparotomy), right iliac fossa (appendicectomy), right upper quadrant (open cholecystectomy), lower abdomen (cesarean section, gynecological procedures), as well as the insertion sites of laparoscopic ports (port-site hernias). With respet to the time of their occurence, the vast majority of incisional hernias occurs within the first 5 years post surgery, stressing the need for extended follow-up of the patients who are at high risk for development of incisional hernias [18]. Incisional hernias at sites of previous hernia repairs can also be described as "recurrent" hernias. Special note should be made to the parastomal hernias and other less common types, such as the semilunar and obturator hernias, which although technically arising from myofascial defects of the anterior trunk, they are traditionally not included in the category of ventral hernias and hence they are not addressed in this chapter.

4. Principles of pre-operative assessment, planning and decision-making

Thorough clinical examination is the first key step in the diagnostic pathway of the patients with ventral hernia. Despite the limitations which can be expected when in comes for instance to the examination of a morbidly obese patient, physical examination is essential to allow an initial estimation of the hernia features, such as size, reducability and presence of multiple defects. Detailed history regarding the relevant symptomatology and accompanying medical comorbidities, as well as previous abdominal operations is critical prior to planning any hernia repair. From a medicolegal point of view, we tend to reserve a minimum of 20-min consultation slot for each new referral in our outpatient clinic, in order to avoid time pressure during the patients' initial assessment. In addition, for "straighforward" cases of ventral hernias (ie small primary defects in fit patients), where the patient can be put directly on the waiting list, we strongly advise that the operating surgeon and the pateint countersign the consent form for the procedure during the visit in the clinic rather than on the day of the actual operation, to ensure mutual understanding of the procedure details and associated risks and implications.

In cases of uncertainity regarding the actual extent of the hernia, presence of multiple subclinical defects, previous failed hernia repairs, as well as in cases where co-existing intra-abdominal pathology warrants exclusion, we strongly advocate for the performance of additional imaging essays of the anterior abdominal wall, with computet tomography (CT) scan being the modality of choice. Anecdotally, in our practice, we tend to almost routinely perform CT scans pre-operatively in all patients with significant size defects, in order to pre-empty the need for implementation of abdominal wall reconstructive adjunct techniques (discussed later), as well as in patients with recurrent incisional hernias, as the clinical examination an easily miss small and subclinical at the time defects. Regarding pre-operative optimisation, smoking cessation is mandatory, due it well-known impact on post-operative wound infections, hernia recurrence rates and pulmonary complications. Especially in cases with major defects, pre-operative consultation by the anaesthesiologist is also sought, so as to correct any outstanding medical issues, in conjuction with the patient's general/family practiioners. Finally, the patients with complex ventral hernias benefit from a pre-habilitation structured intrervention programme including nutritionist, physiotherapist and psychologist, aiding both the physical and mental preparation. Special note should be given to the increased popularity of implemantation of specialist hernia multi-disciplinary team meetings (MDTs), as it happens with the surgical oncology patients' tumor boards [19]. The benefits of these meetings, with the participation of all the medical and allied health professionals who will be involved in the are of complex hernia patients, is the central co-ordination of care, ability to assess the patient and his/her surgical problem through a more holistic approach, ability to involve other surgical specialities in a proactive manner (eg plastic surgeons in cases of abdominal wall reconstructions) and promotion of institutional expertise through continuous monitoring of patient outcomes during the follow-up periods.

5. Principles of technical approaches and operative strategies

Upon identifiation of the clinical need to repair a ventral hernia, the next key questions arise: "open or laparoscopic?", "mesh or primary suture?", "if to use a mesh, where should that be placed?"

With respect to the open versus laparoscopic approach, the expansion of minimally invasive techniques and the attracting concept to the patients has resulted in a significant decrease of the number of ventral hernia cases performed with the traditional open approach. The well-known benefits of laparoscopic surgery, such as reduced hospital stay, improved post-operative pain control, less tissue handling, better cosmesis due to the performance of smaller insicions, have to be considered in ventral hernia repairs [20, 21]. However, one should also bear in mind that laparoscopic surgery has it own natural limitations, like the need for a minimum of three separate incisions (laparoscope, two operating trocars) to perform the procedure, requirement of a medically stable patient who can tolerate the pneumoperitoneum and afford physically a probably longer operative time (excluding essentially the patients with significant co-morbidities or the critically unwell patients with incarcerated-strangulated ventral hernias), absence of extensive intra-abdominal adhesions, which could be the case in patients with incisional hernias and absence of intra-abdominal contamination in particular cases, like the ones with expected need for previous mesh explantation etc. [22]. Obviously, prior laparoscopic surgery experience of the team plays a crucial role here, allowing to "push the envelope" sometimes with undertaking laparoscopic hernia repair in more comple than the average cases. Sometimes though the operating surgeon should bear in mind that the preferrable way is the easiest and fastest one, taking into account that most ventral hernia repairs could be safely performed in the traditional open fashion even by a surgical trainee; hence, complicating a straightforward open case for no reason will potentially just result in avoidable morbidity.

Regarding the use of mesh versus primary suture repair, the globally accepted consensus is that for defects <1 cm primary suture repair is acceptable, while for hernia defects >2 cm the use of prosthetic re-enforcement is advised; for the gray-zone of ventral hernia defects between 1 and 2 cm, an individualized risk/benefit approach is usually followed, balancing between a theoretically higher risk of hernia recurrence versus potential mesh-related complications [23, 24]. At this point, due to the existence of a number of patients who under no circumstances want the insertion of a prosthetic material in their body, the operating surgeon and the patient should have had this relevant discussion during the initial planning consultation and a tissue-only repair is sometimes mandated by the patients' wishes. Another common scenario that detters many surgeons from using mesh and therefore renders the "mesh vs no-mesh" dilemma unnecessary, is the presence of surgical field contamination, although biological meshes could serve as a solution to the problem in cases where augmentation of a simple suture repair is required or as a bridging strategy in patients with loss of domain, where tissue approximation is not deemed possible. The chosen type of mesh can be placed under the subcutaneous tissue layer (onlay), within the myofascial complexes of the abdominal wall (inlay, such as the retro-rectus position), in the preperitoneal space (sublay) or under the parietal peritoneum, in a fully intraperitoneal location [25]. All these anatomical spaces have their pros and cons with respect to hernia recurrence rates, technical ease, seroma formation, occurrence of wound infections/breakdowns. The operating surgeon needs to individualize the repair plan and for instance balance the benefit of a straightforward onlay mesh repair with the known higher chance of wound infections and seromas that accompany this technique.

Probably the key to the success of the repair of ventral hernias is the achievement of a tension-free repair with preservation of the blood and nerve supply to the anterior abdominal wall, as discussed earlier. Although this may be relatively easy with small defects, eg up to 5 cm, in cases of wider defects additional strategies might be required for a tension-free repair. Under this notion, the so-called "component separation techniques", with an anterior and posterior approach have been described. Although detailed description of these techniques exceeds the scope of this chapter, the common concept is that by appropriate division of myofascial elements, the release of the anterior abodminal wall components from their tight investments allows to gain more than 5 cm advancement gain in the epigastric region and a smaller but equally significant myofascial medialisation in the suprapubic region, enabling tension-free closure of large defects [26, 27]. Relatively recently, the "chemical component separation" technique has emerged, using Botox injections to paralyze temporarily the anterior abdominal wall masculature at the level of the forthcoming intervention, in order to allow for a more natural relaxation of the muscles and achievement of tension-free clousre [28]. Finally, in some centers, the use of progressive pneumoperitoneum is utilized, with the patient undergoing sessions of progressive abdominal wall distension, aiming to mecahnically stretch the anterior abdominal wall masculature and facilitate large defects' closure [29].

6. Summary

The management of ventral hernias can be as simple as placement of a few interrupted sutures or as difficult as a formal anterior abdominal wall reconstruction. Careful pre-operative planning with liberal use of appropriate imaging can help to formulate an accurate operative plan and minimize the chance for avoidable complications. The same accounts for the fundamental principle of holistic assessment of the patients and their needs, as well as their expectations. In addition, we strongly advocate routine follow-up of patients who are at high risk of developing incisional hernias, in a similar mindset to the follow-up of patients who undergo curative cancer operations, as early identifcitaion of an incisional/recurrent hernia facilitates its management. Finally, one should always bear in mind that the fact that a hernia operation is at the end of the day an "easy operation" is only a misleading stereotype and complex abdominal wall hernias should be ideally approached by experienced surgeons in centers with an established hernia service, rather than being attempted by novice or inexperienced surgeons.

Author details

Chrysanthi Papageorgopoulou[1], Konstantinos Nikolakopoulos[1], Fotios Efthymiou[2] and Charalampos Seretis[1,3]*

1 Department of General and Vascular Surgery, General University Hospital of Patras, Achaia, Greece

2 Department of Medical Physics, School of Medicine, University of Patras, Achaia, Greece

3 Medical School, University of Warwick, United Kingdom

*Address all correspondence to: babismed@gmail.com

IntechOpen

© 2022 The Author(s). Licensee IntechOpen. This chapter is distributed under the terms of the Creative Commons Attribution License (http://creativecommons.org/licenses/by/3.0), which permits unrestricted use, distribution, and reproduction in any medium, provided the original work is properly cited.

References

[1] Jelinek LA, Scharbach S, Kashyap S, Ferguson T. Anatomy, abdomen and pelvis, anterolateral abdominal wall fascia. In: StatPearls [Internet]. Treasure Island (FL): StatPearls Publishing; 2021

[2] Wright N, Burns B. Anatomy, abdomen and pelvis, posterior abdominal wall arteries. In: StatPearls [Internet]. Treasure Island (FL): StatPearls Publishing; 2021

[3] Ponten JE, Somers KY, Nienhuijs SW. Pathogenesis of the epigastric hernia. Hernia. 2012;**16**(6):627-633. DOI: 10.1007/s10029-012-0964-8

[4] Nassereddin A, Sajjad H. Anatomy, abdomen and pelvis, linea semilunaris. In: StatPearls [Internet]. Treasure Island (FL): StatPearls Publishing; 2021

[5] Seeras K, Qasawa RN, Ju R, Prakash S. Anatomy, abdomen and pelvis, anterolateral abdominal wall. In: StatPearls [Internet]. Treasure Island (FL): StatPearls Publishing; 2021

[6] Sevensma KE, Leavitt L, Pihl KD. Anatomy, abdomen and pelvis, rectus sheath. In: StatPearls [Internet]. Treasure Island (FL): StatPearls Publishing; 2021

[7] Rozen WM, Ashton MW, Taylor GI. Reviewing the vascular supply of the anterior abdominal wall: Redefining anatomy for increasingly refined surgery. Clinical Anatomy. 2008;**21**(2):89-98. DOI: 10.1002/ca.20585

[8] Le Saint-Grant A, Taylor A, Varsou O, Grant C, Cezayirli E, Bowness J. Arterial anatomy of the anterior abdominal wall: Ultrasound evaluation as a real-time guide to percutaneous instrumentation. Clinical Anatomy. 2021;**34**(1):5-10. DOI: 10.1002/ca.23578. Epub 2020 Feb 8

[9] Chin KJ, McDonnell JG, Carvalho B, Sharkey A, Pawa A, Gadsden J. Essentials of our current understanding: Abdominal wall blocks. Regional Anesthesia and Pain Medicine. 2017;**42**(2):133-183. DOI: 10.1097/AAP.0000000000000545

[10] Elhage SA, Marturano MN, Prasad T, Colavita PD, Kercher KW, Augenstein VA, et al. Impact of perforator sparing on anterior component separation outcomes in open abdominal wall reconstruction. Surgical Endoscopy. 2021;**35**(8):4624-4631. DOI: 10.1007/s00464-020-07888-8

[11] Kushner B, Holden S, Blatnik J. Surgical "error traps" of open posterior component separation-transversus abdominis release. Hernia. 2021;**25**(6):1703-1714. DOI: 10.1007/s10029-020-02321-4

[12] Kokotovic D, Sjølander H, Gögenur I, Helgstrand F. Correlation between early surgical complications and readmission rate after ventral hernia repair. Hernia. 2017;**21**(4):563-568. DOI: 10.1007/s10029-017-1606-y

[13] Ponten JE, Somers KY, Nienhuijs SW. Pathogenesis of the epigastric hernia. Hernia. 2012;**16**:627-633

[14] Dufour I, Marique L, Valembois T, Ghilain A, Beniuga G, Tinton N, et al. Ventral primary hernia with liver content. Case Reports in Surgery. 2021;**2021**:6698361. DOI: 10.1155/2021/6698361

[15] Olsson A, Kiwanuka O, Wilhelmsson S, Sandblom G, Stackelberg O. Surgical repair of diastasis recti abdominis provides long-term improvement of abdominal core function and quality of life: A 3-year follow-up.

BJS Open. 2021;**5**(5):zrab085. DOI: 10.1093/bjsopen/zrab085

[16] Almeflh W, AlRaymoony A, AlDaaja MM, Abdullah B, Oudeh A. A systematic review of current consensus on timing of operative repair versus spontaneous closure for asymptomatic umbilical hernias in pediatric. Medical Archives. 2019;**73**(4):268-271. DOI: 10.5455/medarh.2019.73.268-271

[17] Pandya B, Huda T, Gupta D, Mehra B, Narang R. Abdominal wall hernias: An epidemiological profile and surgical experience from a rural medical college in central India. Surgery Journal (NY). 2021;**7**(1):e41-e46. DOI: 10.1055/s-0040-1722744

[18] Dey S, Parthasarathi R, Sabnis SC, Jain R, Praveen Raj P, Senthilnathan P, et al. Laparoscopic management of recurrent ventral hernia: An experience of 222 patients. Hernia. 2019;**23**(5):927-934. DOI: 10.1007/s10029-019-01912-0

[19] Muirhead LJ, Shaw AV, Kontovounisios C, Warren OJ. Establishing a robust multidisciplinary team process in complex abdominal wall reconstruction within a colorectal surgical unit. Techniques in Coloproctology. 2019;**23**(4):379-383. DOI: 10.1007/s10151-019-01965-4

[20] Pereira C, Rai R. Open versus laparoscopic ventral hernia repair: A randomized clinical trial. Cureus. 2021;**13**(12):e20490. DOI: 10.7759/cureus.20490. eCollection 2021 Dec

[21] Al-Taher RN, Khrais IA, Alma'aitah S, Al Saiad AA, Al-Abboodi AA, Saleh OM, et al. Is the open approach superior to the laparoscopic hernia repair in children? A retrospective comparative study. Annals of Medicine and Surgery (London). 2021;**71**:102889. DOI: 10.1016/j.amsu.2021.102889

[22] Cuccurullo D, Piccoli M, Agresta F, Magnone S, Corcione F, Stancanelli V, et al. Laparoscopic ventral incisional hernia repair: Evidence-based guidelines of the first Italian Consensus Conference. Hernia. 2013;**17**(5):557-566. DOI: 10.1007/s10029-013-1055-1

[23] Köckerling F, Brunner W, Fortelny R, Mayer F, Adolf D, Niebuhr H, et al. Treatment of small (<2 cm) umbilical hernias: Guidelines and current trends from the Herniamed Registry. Hernia. 2021;**25**(3):605-617. DOI: 10.1007/s10029-020-02345-w

[24] Henriksen NA, Montgomery A, Kaufmann R, Berrevoet F, East B, Fischer J, et al. Guidelines for treatment of umbilical and epigastric hernias from the European Hernia Society and Americas Hernia Society. The British Journal of Surgery. 2020;**107**(3):171-190. DOI: 10.1002/bjs.11489

[25] Parker SG, Halligan S, Liang MK, Muysoms FE, Adrales GL, Boutall A, et al. International classification of abdominal wall planes (ICAP) to describe mesh insertion for ventral hernia repair. The British Journal of Surgery. 2020;**107**(3):209-217. DOI: 10.1002/bjs.11400

[26] Majumder A, Miller HJ, Del Campo LM, Soltanian H, Novitsky YW. Assessment of myofascial medialization following posterior component separation via transversus abdominis muscle release in a cadaveric model. Hernia. 2018;**22**(4):637-644. DOI: 10.1007/s10029-018-1771-7

[27] Majumder A, Martin-Del-Campo LA, Miller HJ, Podolsky D, Soltanian H, Novitsky YW. Evaluation of anterior versus posterior component separation for hernia repair in a cadaveric model. Surgical Endoscopy.

2020;**34**(6):2682-2689. DOI: 10.1007/s00464-019-07046-9

[28] Zielinski MD, Goussous N, Schiller HJ, Jenkins D. Chemical components separation with botulinum toxin A: A novel technique to improve primary fascial closure rates of the open abdomen. Hernia. 2013;**17**(1):101-107. DOI: 10.1007/s10029-012-0995-1

[29] Van Rooijen MMJ, Yurtkap Y, Allaeys M, Ibrahim N, Berrevoet F, Lange JF. Fascial closure in giant ventral hernias after preoperative botulinum toxin a and progressive pneumo peritoneum: A systematic review and meta-analysis. Surgery. 2021;**170**(3):769-776. DOI: 10.1016/j.surg.2021.03.027

Chapter 3

Totally Extraperitoneal Approach (TEP) for Inguinal Hernia Repair

Ioannis Triantafyllidis

Abstract

Laparoscopic inguinal herniorrhaphy was initially described by Ger in the early 1980s. Nowadays, two techniques are worldwide adopted: the transabdominal preperitoneal approach (TAPP) and the totally extraperitoneal approach (TEP). In these repairs, the myopectineal orifice is approached posteriorly and allows for inguinal, femoral, and obturator hernia repairs to be performed simultaneously. TEP is a relatively new technique. McKernan and Law first introduced TEP in 1993. Some proponents of TEP advocate for this technique over the transabdominal approach due to the shorter operative times, especially for bilateral hernias, and decrease the risks of vascular, bowel, and bladder injuries as well as bowel obstructions, adhesions, or fistula formation potentially associated with intraperitoneal dissection and intraperitoneal mesh exposure. When compared with open hernia repair, and in particular for recurrent (after open) and bilateral hernias, many surgeons prefer the laparoendoscopic approach due to quicker recovery times and less postoperative and chronic pain. In experienced hands, there are no absolute contraindications to TEP, although a careful decision should be made to tailor the approach to both patient and surgeon factors. In this chapter, we will describe the technical steps of totally extraperitoneal hernia repair, the potential complications, and troubleshooting when needed.

Keywords: hernia repair, inguinal, totally extraperitoneal, laparoendoscopic, myopectineal orifice, mesh

1. Introduction

Repair of groin hernia is one of the most common elective operations performed in general surgical practice. Bassini's [1] sutured repair became a milestone in the repair of groin hernia. Lichtenstein [2] popularized the tension-free open mesh repair using polypropylene mesh claiming rapid ambulation and recovery with a 99% probability of permanent cure. Minimal access approaches to inguinal hernia repair have added to the ongoing debate over the best groin hernia repair [3, 4]. Ger and associates [5] in 1990 introduced laparoscopic inguinal hernia repair. The current concept of laparoscopic repair is based on Stoppa's [6] concept of preperitoneal reinforcement of fascia transversalis over the myopectineal orifice with a large piece of mesh. In 2004, the National Institute of Health and Clinical Excellence

(NICE) [7] published guidelines after a meta-analysis of over 40 randomized controlled trials and reported that laparoscopic repair was indeed associated with less pain and faster recovery, but also with increased cost and longer operating times and that laparoscopic surgery is considered as one of the treatment options for the repair of inguinal hernia. There are two standardized laparoscopic techniques: transabdominal preperitoneal approach (TAPP) described by Arregui et al. [8] in the early 1990s and totally extraperitoneal approach (TEP) described by Mckernon and Laws [9] in 1993.

TEP laparoscopic inguinal hernia repair has gained popularity in the past few years and is preferred over TAPP repair as it is less invasive and avoids entry to the peritoneal cavity. TEP procedure combines the advantages of minimal invasive surgery and those of tension-free mesh repair. TEP is a complex procedure that is performed in a space created during operation. It is necessary to be skilled in laparoscopic surgery and familiar with the anatomy of the abdominal wall from within to perform the operation with good results. During the learning curve, one of the difficulties is finding the correct plane in the preperitoneal space. If dissection is performed in the wrong surgical plane, there is increased risk of hemorrhage, loss of anatomical plane, or both. Laparoendoscopic inguinal hernia repair when compared with open approaches in various trials, either randomized or prospective, revealed significant benefits and advantageous outcomes, such as less postoperative pain, faster recovery and return to physical activity, as well as superior cosmesis [10, 11]. Furthermore, during laparoendoscopic hernia repair, the surgeon has the ability to inspect the entire myopectineal orifice and evaluate the presence of other types of hernia, such as a femoral hernia, which may be repaired in the same procedure [12, 13]. Although, a variety of laparoendoscopic techniques have been described for the management of groin hernias [14–19]; two among them are the most popular regarding inguinal hernioplasty: TAPP and TEP repair. In both methods, a mesh prosthesis is implanted into the preperitoneal space dorsal to the transversalis fascia. These techniques therefore represent minimally invasive versions of open mesh implantation techniques. In TAPP, the surgeon enters the peritoneal cavity and places a mesh through a peritoneal incision over possible hernia sites. TEP is superior because the peritoneal cavity is not entered and mesh is used to seal the hernia from outside the peritoneum. This approach is considered to be more difficult than TAPP but may result in fewer complications. The TAPP approach has been advocated for complicated hernias (sliding or incarcerated inguinal hernias) and hernias with previous pelvic surgery (radical prostatectomy). This technique has been criticized for exposing intraabdominal organs to potential complications, including small bowel injury and obstruction. Laparoscopic TEP hernia repair has gained ground in recent years and is preferred over TAPP as it is less invasive and is associated with fewer complications. In their comparative study, Felix et al. reported 11 major complications in the TAPP group (two recurrences, six hernias in the trocar site, and others), whereas only one recurrence was observed in the TEP group, with no intraperitoneal complications [14]. Khoury et al. found that patients who underwent TEP received less narcotic analgesia than those who underwent TAPP and that they were discharged more frequently at the operative day [20]. Although, traditionally, open hernia repair was favored over laparoendoscopic repairs, as far as cost-effectiveness is concerned [21, 22], nowadays, it seems that in a cost analysis context, TEP is comparable with conventional open repair [23, 24]. Taking into account that in experienced surgeons, operating time and morbidity, especially recurrences, are significantly reduced, laparoendoscopic inguinal hernia repair techniques became more popular, and more and more surgeons favor them for most types of inguinal hernias. Furthermore, more surgeons prefer TEP over TAPP because the peritoneal cavity is not entered and in such a way less intraabdominal complications may occur.

2. Anatomy of the inguinal preperitoneal space

The preperitoneal space lies between the peritoneum and the posterior lamina of the transversalis fascia. There are two important spaces in the setting of laparoendoscopic inguinal hernia repair: the space of Retzius, the most medial of which lies superior to the bladder, and the space of Bogros, which is a lateral extension of the space of Retzius that extends to the level of the anterior superior iliac spine. Dissection of these spaces gives the surgeon access to the myopectineal orifice of Fruchaud, which is bound superiorly by the aponeurotic arch of the internal oblique and the transversus abdominis muscle, inferiorly by the Cooper ligament, medially by the lateral border of the rectus muscle, and laterally by the iliopsoas muscle. The inguinal ligament and iliopubic tract pass obliquely through this space (**Figure 1**).

Three potential sites of hernia formation are associated with the myopectineal orifice: the indirect, the direct, and the femoral space. The direct and indirect spaces are located medial and lateral to the inferior epigastric vessels, respectively, and both are

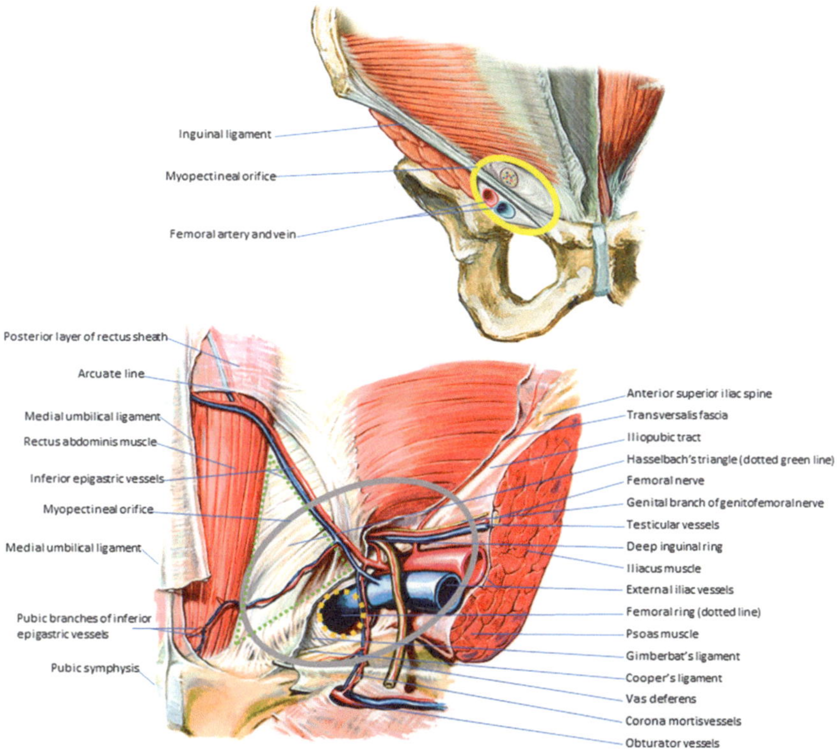

Figure 1.
Anterior and posterior views of myopectineal orifice (from Elliott and Novitsky [25]).

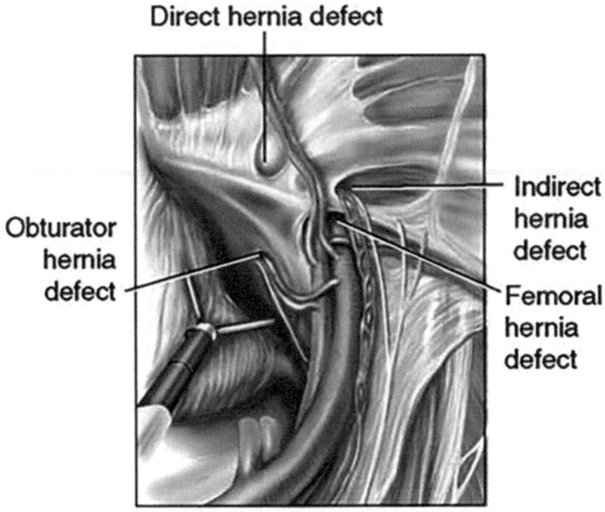

Figure 2.
Potential hernia sites within the myopectineal orifice (direct, indirect, obturator, and femoral). Placement of mesh over entire myopectineal orifice. Usually, no stapling devices are used for placement of mesh.

above the iliopubic tract. The femoral canal lies in the area bounded anterosuperiorly by the inguinal ligament, posteriorly by the pectineal ligament lying anterior to the superior pubic ramus, medially by the lacunar ligament, and laterally by the femoral vein (**Figure 2**).

Furthermore, three triangles are important in laparoscopic hernia repair: Hesselbach's triangle with its' medial border consisted of the lateral margin of the rectus sheath, the superolateral border defined by the inferior epigastric vessels, whereas the inferior border is the Poupart ligament, the "triangle of Doom" bordered medially by the vas deferens and laterally by the vessels of the spermatic cord, with its base opposite to the deep ring (the contents of this space include the external iliac vessels, deep circumflex iliac vein, femoral nerve, and genital branch of the genitofemoral nerve) and the "triangle of Pain," which is bounded by the gonadal vessels medially, the reflected peritoneum laterally, and the iliopubic tract superiorly (the femoral nerve, the genitofemoral nerve, the anterior femoral cutaneous nerve, and the lateral femoral cutaneous nerve are found in this region).

3. Indications and contraindications

It is generally accepted that laparoscopic inguinal hernia repair is indicated for bilateral hernias or recurrent following open repair [26]. The laparoendoscopic approach avoids the morbidity associated with bilateral groin incisions and allows for bilateral repair with one operation. Furthermore, it obviates the necessity to dissect in the anterior plane where the surgical field may be jeopardized from previous repairs, especially if a mesh has been used. Increasingly, surgeons have been offering laparoscopic repair upfront, even in the setting of unilateral, previously unrepaired hernias due to the reduction in postoperative acute pain and time away from work and daily activities, as well overall improved quality of life [27].

This is particularly true for surgeons who are familiar and have experienced the laparoendoscopic technique. Surgeons during their early experience should preferably operate on thin patients fit for general anesthesia with small, direct, uncomplicated, or indirect reducible hernias.

Although there are no absolute contraindications to totally extraperitoneal hernia repair in the elective setting, apart from patient's inability to tolerate general anesthesia or pneumoperitoneum due to cardiopulmonary disease, previous pelvic irradiation or surgery, lower midline or ipsilateral paramedian incisions, large inguinoscrotal or chronically irreducible hernias as well as recurrent hernias from a previous TEP are relative contraindications. With the blind balloon dissection required for the TEP technique, there is a risk of injury to the contents of the incarcerated hernia sac. Extraperitoneal endoscopic repair is difficult and time-consuming in these circumstances. In these instances, one may elect to attempt a TAPP repair and convert to the open operation if it is obvious that this, too, is not feasible. Modifications from a traditional TEP should include mandatory Foley catheter placement to allow for full development of the space of Retzius as well as surgeon comfort with ligating the epigastric vessels, if needed, as well as knowledge on how to incise the transversalis fascial sling to aid in indirect hernia sac reduction [28]. Previous appendectomy is usually not a problem, but the surgeon should be more careful during the lateral dissection. Acute abdomen with strangulated and/or infected inguinal hernias that will require bowel resection and pediatric patients are absolute contraindications.

4. Preoperative planning and patient preparation

A complete history and physical examination are mandatory to assess the patient's fitness for general anesthesia. The patient is examined while standing and supine for both inguinal and femoral hernias on both left and right sides. A preoperative imaging with ultrasonography or computed tomography is justified to rule out any doubt in the diagnosis of the inguinal hernia. Special measures must be taken if the patient is on drugs such as anticoagulants; if the patient is on acetylsalicylic acid and related drugs (these must be discontinued at least a week before surgery); and if the patient is on oral warfarin (should be placed on heparin or its long-acting derivatives). A pre-anesthetic check-up must be done to get clearance for surgery.

The patient should be informed that there is a risk of conversion to TAPP or to an open approach depending on the difficulty and the safety of the procedure. Any possible complications such as vascular or nerve injuries, mesh infection, chronic postoperative pain, hematoma, seroma or injury to the spermatic cord, bowel and urinary bladder, as well as risks from CO_2 insufflation (hypotension, hypercapnea, subcutaneous emphysema, etc.), should be thoroughly explained to the patient [29].

Prophylactic antibiotic administration such as a single dose of a first-generation cephalosporin before the induction of anesthesia is recommended in the presence of risk factors for wound and mesh infection, such as advanced age, steroid use, obesity, diabetes mellitus, immunosuppression, malignancy, prolonged operating time and/or insertion of drains [30, 31]. Umbilical disinfection is recommended, and possibly shaving or depilation from the umbilicus halfway down to the symphysis. The patient should have emptied their bladder shortly before surgery and a catheter is not necessary, unless the operation takes more than 1.5 h. No bowel preparation is necessary. All patients undergoing totally extraperitoneal hernia repair receive deep vein thrombosis prophylaxis.

5. Anesthesia

Totally extraperitoneal hernia repair may be performed using local, epidural, or general anesthesia. Many surgeons find that spinal anesthesia is adequate for the TEP repair most of the time. Rarely, especially if the peritoneum is breached, conversion to general anesthesia may be required. However, it is our preference to operate under general anesthesia, because this type of anesthesia ensures that any cardiovascular or respiratory effect of CO_2 insufflation is minimized. Furthermore these effects are comparable to those attributed to intraperitoneal CO_2 insufflation [32].

6. Suggested equipment

- A 5- or 10-mm, 0° or 30° angled laparoscope
- A 5- or 10-mm Hasson's trocar for the laparoscope
- One balloon/space-making trocar (optional; based on the International Endohernia Society guidelines, it is recommended to use a balloon dissector when creating the preperitoneal space, especially during the learning curve, when it is difficult to identify the correct preperitoneal plane and space [31])
- Two 5-mm trocars
- Two 5-mm fenestrated grasping forceps
- A 5-mm strong grasping forceps
- Monopolar energy device and cable
- A pair of dissecting and coagulating shears
- Scissors
- Laparoscopic clips (5 mm)
- A 5-mm endoscopic needle holder
- A Verres needle
- Synthetic mesh (i.e., a preshaped 3-D polypropylene mesh) (size may vary i.e., 15 × 10 cm or 17 × 12 cm)
- A suction cannula
- Endoloops
- Tackers and fixation devices

7. Technical considerations

7.1 Operating room setup

The patient is placed, under—usually—general anesthesia, in the supine position, with the arm on the side of the hernia extended, although many surgeons prefer both arms to be tucked. It is helpful to put the patient in a 15° Trendelenburg position. The monitor is positioned at the foot end of the patient. The surgeon stands on the side opposite of the hernia and the camera operator (assistant) and the scrub nurse at the side of the hernia.

7.2 Extraperitoneal access, trocar placement, and dissection of the preperitoneal space

We have adopted Dulucq's [33] technique and a Veress needle is initially inserted above the pubis in the midline in order to penetrate the linea alba (**Figure 3**). The needle enters the preperitoneal space and is inserted in the Retzius space, which is insufflated with 2 lit of CO_2. This initial "pneumodissection" of Retzius space facilitates the insertion of the working trocars and further dissection of the surgical planes. After the insufflation of CO_2, a 1 cm periumbilical incision, ipsilateral to the hernia is made and the anterior rectus sheath is incised at the level of arcuate line, a point roughly level with the anterior superior iliac spine, and a 10-mm trocar is inserted into the preperitoneal space. The laparoscope is then introduced and the space is progressively expanded by blunt telescope dissection with a 0° or 30° laparoscope and CO_2 insufflation at a continuous pressure of 12 mmHg. Alternatively, a dissecting balloon may be used to save time and facilitate the creation of the space, but this is not mandatory while it increases the cost of the procedure. Gentle side-to-side movements of the

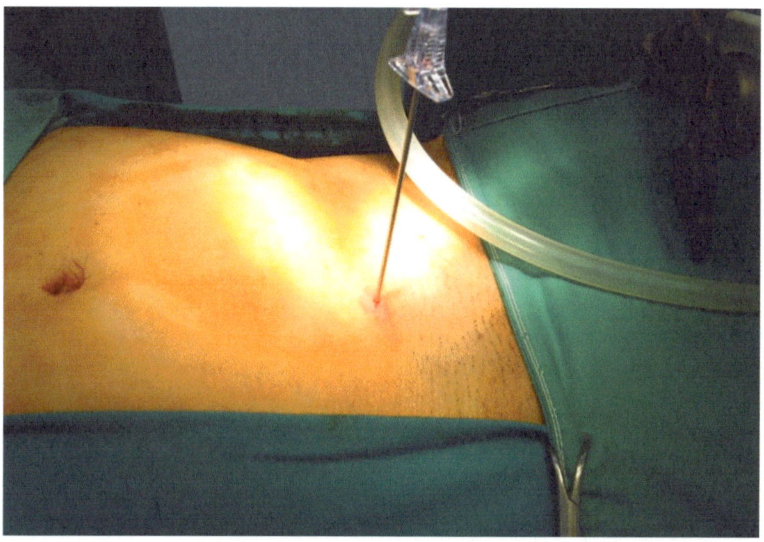

Figure 3.
A Veress needle is initially inserted above the pubis in the midline in order to penetrate the linea alba. The needle enters the preperitoneal space and is inserted in the Retzius space, which is insufflated with 2 l of CO_2.

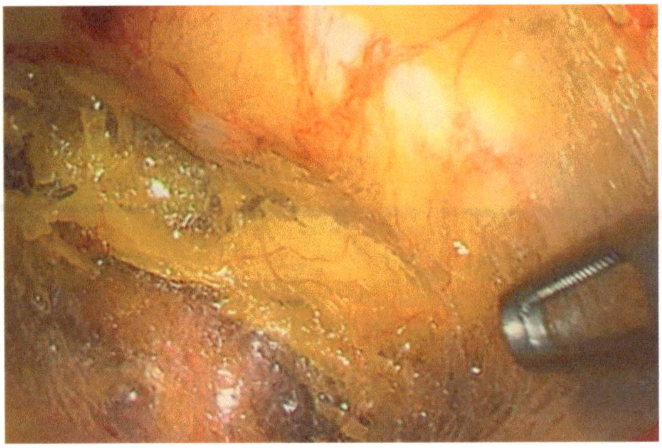

Figure 4.
Cooper's ligament is the first anatomical landmark of our dissection and appears as a white glistening structure.

laparoscope are used to dissect the areolar tissue. The inferior epigastric vessels are clearly visualized laterally on the posterior surface of the rectus muscle, and special care is taken not to injure them to avoid an unpleasant intraoperative bleeding that may be difficult to control. The retropubic space of Retzius and the space of Bogros are easily expanded by the telescopic approach and under direct view a 5-mm working trocar is introduced in the midline, midway between the umbilicus and pubic symphysis. Thereafter, the preperitoneal space is widened by sharp and blunt dissection under direct view and a second working trocar is placed two finger breadths medially to the superior anterior iliac spine on the side of the hernia, thereby respecting the triangulation principle and allowing adequate lateral mesh placement. An alternative is to place both working trocars in the infraumbilical midline, a setup that allows bilateral inguinal repair with the same trocars, although it makes dissection more difficult due to the lack of triangulation. The lower border of the pubic bone and Cooper's ligament should be exposed, noting the iliac vein and structures of the obturator foramen. This is the first anatomical landmark and appears as a white glistening structure (**Figure 4**). The space beyond the symphysis pubis is exposed for 2–3 cm to the obturator fossa, thus allowing the medial lower placement of the mesh. Extra care should be paid to avoid an injury in the urinary bladder. An injury to corona mortis at this stage should be avoided at all costs, as an intractable and uncontrollable hemorrhage may occur. Moving toward the anterior superior iliac spine in a surgical plane that is below the inferior epigastric vessels and above the peritoneum, the lateral dissection is made by pushing down the peritoneum until the psoas muscle can be seen. The space of Bogros is delineated and cleaned all the way up to the anterior superior iliac spine. Attention should be paid to avoid dissecting further laterally, in the so-called "triangle of pain." This will prevent injury to the latero-cutaneous and genitofemoral nerves. Once the medial and lateral dissection is completed, the surgeon is able to identify the entire hernia defect, followed by a proper hernia sac reduction and repair.

7.3 Dissection of hernial sac

The hernia sac is gradually dissected by gentle traction on the cord elements to identify and free the peritoneal sac from the spermatic cord, vas deferens, and spermatic vessels. It is useful to isolate the hernial sac from the spermatic cord close

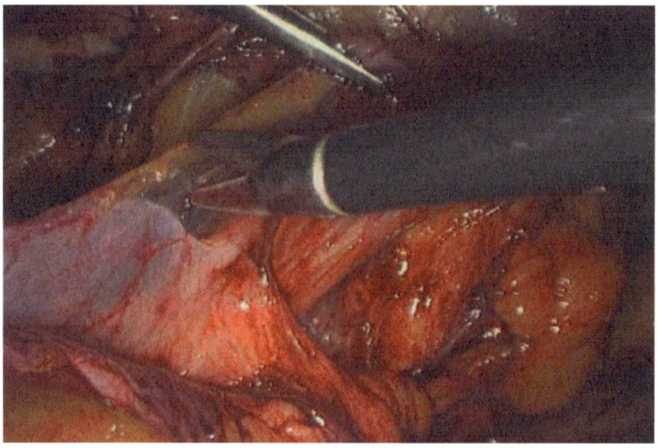

Figure 5.
Indirect hernia sac dissection.

to the deep inguinal ring, approaching from the lateral side, and then mobilize it from the inguinal canal by blunt dissection [31]. A large hernia sac may be left reverted inside the peritoneal cavity without resection. However, it can also be divided at the deep ring; this is strongly recommended for larger lateral hernias as extensive dissection may result in scrotal edema and postoperative pain. Such a sac should be separated from the cord, ligated (i.e., with an endo-loop), and divided distal to the ligature leaving the distal part of the sac open. A direct hernia sac is easily dissected bluntly from the transversalis fascia by simple traction, inverted, and anchored to the Cooper's ligament with a suture or a clip to prevent a seroma formation or a pseudo-recurrence. The peritoneum is pushed back as far as possible into the abdominal cavity. The anterior part of the psoas muscle, as well as the crossing of the iliac vein by the vas deferens, must be fully exposed [33]. Laterally, the peritoneal sac is mobilized posteriorly at least 5 cm from the inguinal ligament usually possible without sharp dissection. The cord should be completely skeletonized to the extent where the vas deferens is seen turning medially. This maneuver exposes the "triangle of Doom." Dissection should be avoided within this triangle. A lipoma is often present in the inguinal canal and ideally should be resected or at least completely reduced. In case of bilateral hernias, the surgeon and camera assistant change sides and a similar dissection is performed on the opposite side (**Figure 5**).

A lateral hernia is usually found in females, and in such cases, skeletonization of the round ligament may result in injury of the peritoneum. It is important to close all peritoneal holes with absorbable suture loops or clips to prevent any internal herniation or adhesion formation with the mesh. It is advisable that the round ligament should be divided at the level of the deep inguinal ring between clips because of the arteries within it.

The sac in femoral hernias is reduced by gentle traction with fenestrated forceps. Widening of the femoral defect by using a hook diathermy at its medial-superior aspect in cases of small-sized defects may be necessary to facilitate the hernia sac reduction. An obturator hernia sac may be reduced in the same manner by gentle traction.

7.4 Mesh preparation and placement

Once the anatomic elements are properly identified, including dissection of the peritoneum covering the floor of the anterior pelvic wall, the final step is the hernia

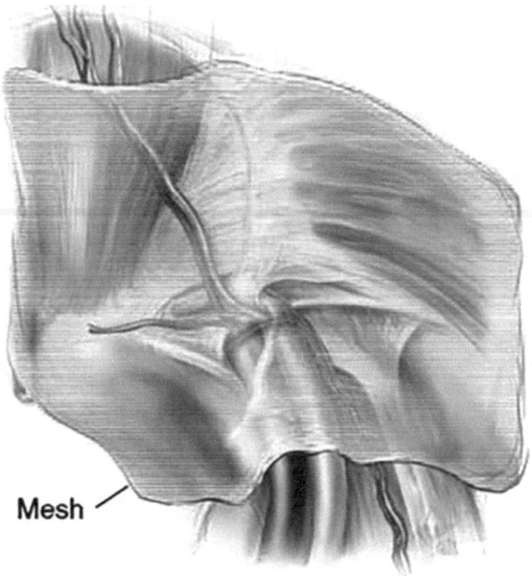

Figure 6.
The ideal mesh should cover all areas of potential herniation, and it should cross the midline for at least 2–3 cm.

repair, which is achieved by covering and reinforcing the entire myopectineal orifice with a suitable mesh. A preshaped 3-D anatomical mesh or a synthetic large-pore prosthesis at least 15 × 11 cm may be used. The ideal mesh should cover all areas of potential herniation, and it should cross the midline for at least 2–3 cm (**Figure 6**). Usually, a 15 × 11 cm mesh is appropriate for a patient with average body habitus. Large hernias will require even larger meshes of 15 × 15 cm. In cases of bilateral hernias, two meshes should be inserted overlapping each other in the midline for at least 3 cm. However, placement of only a large mesh seems a reasonable alternative, although not widely adopted.

A "no-touch technique" is mandatory to avoid mesh infection. Changing glove before handling the mesh is a wise precaution. The mesh is rolled and introduced through the 10 mm umbilical trocar into the preperitoneal cavity avoiding any contact with the skin. The mesh is then placed horizontally and unrolled over the myopectineal orifice making sure to cover sufficiently all potential hernia sites in the inguinal region. One-third of the mesh should be below the symphysis pubis and the upper margin reaching the lower trocar medially. The mesh is placed in the preperiotneal space of Bogros and Retzius in such a way that the inferior edge of the mesh is on the psoas muscle and the lateral edge close to the anterior superior iliac spine, whereas the medial and inferior aspect of the mesh is placed under Cooper's ligament. The inferior edge of the mesh covers the spermatic cord, the vas deferens, and the iliac vessels, while the superior aspect of the mesh is against the rectus and transversus abdominis muscles. It is important to make sure that no part of the peritoneum is under the mesh to prevent any recurrence.

Unlike TAPP, the mesh is usually placed without fixation, and after hemostasis has been achieved, the CO_2 is deflated under vision to ensure that the mesh is not rolled. Folds or wrinkles in the mesh should be avoided because they lead to increased scar or adhesion formation and can be the cause of chronic pain in the future [26]. The lateral inferior edge of the mesh can be held with a grasper, if necessary, especially in cases of bilateral hernias. However, many surgeons prefer to anchor the mesh, with means such as tackers, sealants, or sutures, to prevent mesh migration and associated

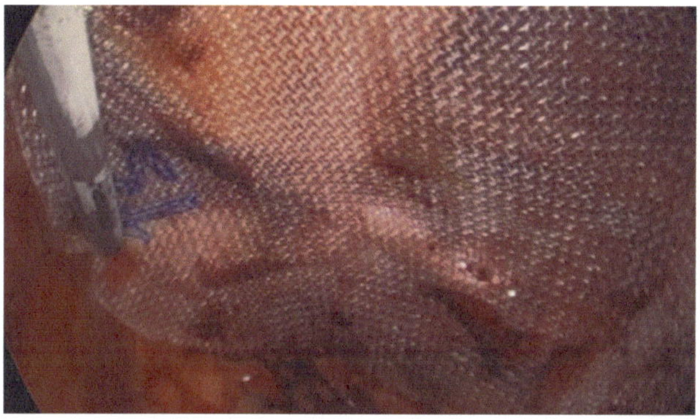

Figure 7.
Fixation of the mesh on Cooper's ligament with tackers.

recurrences. Fixation is usually done on Cooper's ligament, medial to the inferior epigastric vessels at the rectus muscle and, if necessary, lateral to the inferior epigastric vessels (**Figure 7**). Placement of tackers below the iliopubic tract and too laterally considering should be avoided. However, in cases of large direct or femoral hernias, it is advisable to fix the inferior edge of the mesh, either with stapler or sutures, to the pectineal ligament to prevent any slippage into the defect. Drainage of the extraperitoneal space is required rarely, mainly after sharp dissection of adhesions in the surgical field. If carbon dioxide is trapped within the peritoneal cavity, it is evacuated with a Veress needle, inserted at Palmer's point. The ports are then removed and the anterior rectus sheath incision at the 10-mm trocar site is sutured. Gas trapped in the scrotum can also be evacuated by gentle pressure on the scrotum to push the gas into the preperitoneal space and then evacuate through the umbilical port or with a small needle at the end of the procedure, if this is necessary. The skin incisions are then closed with sutures, clips, or glue.

8. Postoperative care

Totally extraperitoneal hernia repair is usually performed under general anesthesia and thus a postoperative surveillance for at least 3–5 h is mandatory before discharge, once voiding freely and if they are hemodynamically stable and normal. Analgesics such as paracetamol or non-steroidal anti-inflammatory drugs are given either through oral route or as rectal suppositories for 2–3 days, if necessary. Diet is resumed as tolerated. Generally, no restrictions are placed upon the patients, and they are allowed to resume physical activity and return to work as soon as their pain tolerance allows them to do so.

9. Complications

Serious intraoperative complications specific to TEP are less frequent than with TAPP [30], occur in about 4–6% of the cases, and can be due to injury to vascular, visceral, nerve, and spermatic cord structures [34].

Vascular injuries would include injury to the external iliac vessels, inferior epigastric or spermatic vessels or the vessels over the pubic, arch including the corona mortis vessels. The most frequent cause of hemorrhage is injury of the epigastric vessels and their branches during extraperitoneal dissection and usually is controlled by clips and/or coagulation with bipolar shears. The lateral or anterior parietal perforating vessels may be controlled by coagulation. However, caution is required during electrocautery in the vicinity of nerves. Bleeding from corona mortis, which represents an anastomosis between the external iliac or the inferior epigastric and the obturator arteries, may occur during the medial dissection in approximately 1.5–2% of cases and results in significant bleeding that may lead to retroperitoneal hematoma, conversion to open or reoperation [35]. The iliac vein can be mistaken for an irreducible hernia and injured, thus necessitating conversion to laparotomy. Injury to the major vessels is catastrophic, a correct lateral traction of the sac and spermatic structure with medial approach may be helpful in avoiding it. A careful practice should be used when retracting or dissecting closer to the "triangle of doom."

Previous lower abdominal surgery poses a risk to injuries of the urinary bladder especially during midline adhesiolysis. The incidence of such a complication is reported to be less than 0.3% [36]. When identified, should be repaired endoscopically and a urinary catheter should be left in the bladder for a week [31]. This type of injury is not an absolute contraindication for mesh implantation.

Bowel injuries may occur during reduction of irreducible hernias or lateral adhesiolysis or as a result of transmitted energy through the thin peritoneal layer. It is mandatory to detect and manage them intraoperatively.

Nerve injuries, usually of the genitofemoral nerve and/or lateral cutaneous nerve of the thigh, and the intermediate cutaneous branch of the femoral nerve occur intraoperatively due to entrapment of the nerve when tacks are used to fix the mesh, thermal injury caused by excessive use of electrocoagulation or irritation caused directly by the mesh. This type of injuries become apparent postoperatively resulting in neuralgia, usually transient. To minimize the incidence of these injuries, one should maintain the correct plane of dissection, which means that the fascia over the psoas muscle should stay intact and the mesh should only be fixed medially, avoiding the "triangle of pain." Knowledge of the groin anatomy is of paramount importance in avoiding nerve injury. Immediate postoperative neuralgia should ideally be managed by re-exploration and removal of the offending tack or piece of mesh. Symptoms of nerve injury usually resolve within 8 weeks. Chronic pain, defined as pain that persists after 3 months, may require prolonged injections with local anesthetic and corticosteroids and rehabilitation and in most severe cases exploration and removal of tacks or a neurectomy [37].

Peritoneal tears may occur in up to 47% of cases [38], resulting in pneumoperitoneum, which diminishes the working space and increases the difficulty of the procedure. Small holes do not need to be repaired. In case of an inadvertent opening of the peritoneum, the pressure drops but the operation usually can go on, if a Verres needle or an intraperitoneal trocar fitted with a valve is required to balance the pressures. If a balance cannot be obtained, the peritoneal opening must be closed with a suture or a clip. The peritoneal repair must be performed either during or at the end of surgery [26, 33].

Seroma and hematoma are the commonest complications following any type of hernia repair. Seroma has a reported incidence of 5–7% after laparoscopic repair, while the incidence of hematoma is around 8%. This, in fact, may mimic a recurrence, but resolves in 90% of patients by 6 weeks. These collections should not be aspirated or drained without obvious signs of infection, unless they cause discomfort and pain, especially if they persist more than 6 weeks, and it appears that they are not resolving. Aspiration should be performed under strict aseptic conditions and may be repeated

2–3 times. Physical examination alone usually establishes the diagnosis and no further imaging modalities are necessary. Careful dissection and hemostasis can help to reduce the incidence of postoperative hematoma [39]. It is important to counsel the patients regarding this complication to avoid fear and unnecessary visits to the emergency department and/or unnecessary imaging studies [39, 40].

Recurrence is one of the most important outcomes of hernia repair. Well-defined parameters that contribute to recurrence are surgeon inexperience, inadequate dissection of the myopectineal orifice, inadequate fixation of the mesh, insufficient mesh size, and failure to cover unidentified hernia defects, mesh folding that allows peritoneal slippage and mesh dislodgement secondary to hematoma formation [34]. There is no evidence that fixation of the mesh affects recurrence rates. A crucial step in preventing recurrence is creating a space wide enough for the mesh to overlap all possible sites of herniation with complete coverage of the myopectineal orifice.

10. Conclusions

Several trials and meta-analyses have shown that TEP is a procedure that carries an acceptable low complication rate and low recurrence rate with the advantages of minimally invasive surgery, when performed by experienced surgeons. Thus, it is associated with reduced postoperative pain, less need for postoperative analgesia, earlier resume of physical activities, and fewer recurrences in comparison to open inguinal hernia repair [31]. These benefits will be exaggerated when the laparoendoscopic technique is implemented in cases of bilateral or recurrent hernias. However, we should take into account that careful patient selection, precise knowledge of the anatomy, an adequate surgical technique, and the surgeon's experience and expertise are the cornerstones of the best clinical outcome with low morbidity. In such a way laparoendoscopic inguinal hernia repair is the procedure of choice for the management of primary and the vast majority of recurrent inguinal hernias.

Conflict of interest

Dr. Ioannis Triantafyllidis declares no conflict of interest.

Abbreviations

TAPP transabdominal preperitoneal approach
TEP totally extraperitoneal approach

Author details

Ioannis Triantafyllidis
Department of Surgery, General Hospital of Kavala, Kavala, Greece

*Address all correspondence to: jtrianta@gmail.com

IntechOpen

© 2022 The Author(s). Licensee IntechOpen. This chapter is distributed under the terms of the Creative Commons Attribution License (http://creativecommons.org/licenses/by/3.0), which permits unrestricted use, distribution, and reproduction in any medium, provided the original work is properly cited.

References

[1] Bassini E. Nuovo metodo sulla cura radicale dell'erniainguinale. Arch Soc Ital Chir 4:380. Basic features of groin hernia and its repair by Sathyaprasad C, Burjonrappa, Samuel Gemaj, Robert J Fitzgibbons Jr. In: Yeo CJ, Gross SD, editors. Shackelford's Surgery of the Alimentary Tract. 6th ed. Amsterdam, Netherlands: Saunders-Elsevier; 1887, 2007. pp. 632-655

[2] Lichtenstein IL, Shulman AG, Amid PK, Montllor MM. The tension-free hernioplasty. American Journal of Surgery. 1989;**157**(2):188-193

[3] The MRC Laparoscopic Groin Hernia Trial Group. Laparoscopic versus open repair of groin hernia: A randomized comparison. Lancet. 1999;**354**(9174):185-190

[4] Neumayer L, Giobbie-Hurder A, Jonasson O, Fitzgibbons R Jr, Dunlop D, Gibbs J, et al. Open mesh versus laparoscopic mesh repair of inguinal hernia. The New England Journal of Medicine. 2004;**350**(18):1819-1827

[5] Ger R, Monroe K, Duvivier R, Mishrick A. Management of indirect inguinal hernias by laparoscopic closure of the neck of the sac. American Journal of Surgery. 1990;**159**(4):370-373

[6] Stoppa RE, Warlaumont CR, Verhaeghe PJ, Romero ER, M'Balla-N'Di CJ. Prosthetic repair in the treatment of groin hernias. International Surgery. 1986;**71**(3):154-158

[7] Laparoscopic Surgery for Inguinal Hernia Repair: Guidance on the Use of. Technology Appraisal Guidance 83, Issue date: September 2004, Review date: September 2007. National Institute for Clinical Excellence. London. WC1V 6NA. Available from: http://www.nice.org.uk/TA083guidance

[8] Arregui ME, Davis CJ, Yucel O, Nagan RF. Laparoscopic mesh repair of inguinal hernia using a preperitoneal approach: A preliminary report. Surgical Laparoscopy & Endoscopy. 1992;**2**(1):53-58

[9] McKernan JB, Laws HL. Laparoscopic repair of inguinal hernias using a totally extraperitoneal prosthetic approach. Surgical Endoscopy. 1993;**7**(1):26-28

[10] Heikkinen TJ, Haukipuro K, Koivukangas P, et al. A prospective randomized outcome and cost comparison of totally extra-peritoneal endoscopic hernioplasty versus Lichtenstein operation among employed patients. Surgical Laparoscopy & Endoscopy. 1998;**8**:338-344

[11] Pawanindra L, Kajla RK, Chander J, et al. Randomized controlled study of laparoscopic total extra-peritoneal versus open Lichtenstein inguinal hernia repair. Surgical Endoscopy. 2003;**17**:850-856

[12] Barrat C, Surlin V, Bordia A, et al. Management of recurrent inguinal hernias: A prospective study of 163 cases. Hernia. 2003;**7**:125-129

[13] Sayad P, Ferzli G. Laparoscopic preperitoneal repair of recurrent inguinal hernias. Journal of Laparoendoscopic & Advanced Surgical Techniques. Part A. 1999;**9**(2):127-130

[14] Camps J, Nguyen N, Annabali R, et al. Laparoscopic inguinal herniorrhaphy: Transabdominal techniques. International Surgery. 1995;**80**:18-25

[15] Felix EL, Michas CA, Gonzalez MH Jr. Laparoscopic hernioplasty: TAPP vs. TEP. Surgical Endoscopy. 1995;**9**:984-989

[16] Sosa JL, Puente I, Markley M, et al. A modified technique of laparoscopic herniorrhaphy: Operative approach and early results. International Surgery. 1994;**79**:300-303

[17] Wishart GC, Wright D, O'Dwyer PJ. Use of a Foley catheter to dissect the preperitoneal space for extraperitoneal endoscopic hernia repair. Journal of Laparoendoscopic Surgery. 1995;**5**:27-29

[18] Dulucq JL. Treatment of inguinal hernias by insertion of mesh through retroperitoneoscopy. Post Graduate General Surgery. 1992;**4**:173-174

[19] Dulucq JL. Pre-peritoneal approach in laparoscopic treatment of inguinal hernia. Journal de Chirurgie. 2000;**137**(5):285-288

[20] Khoury N. A comparative study of laparoscopic extraperitoneal and transabdominal preperitoneal herniorrhaphy. Journal of Laparoendoscopic Surgery. 1995;**5**:349-355

[21] Medical Research Council Laparoscopic Groin Hernia Trial Group. Cost–utility analysis of open versus laparoscopic groin hernia repair: Results from a multicentre randomized clinical trial. The British Journal of Surgery. 2001;**88**:653-661

[22] Liem MS, Halsema JA, van der Graaf Y, et al. Cost effectiveness of extraperitoneal laparoscopic inguinal hernia repair: A randomized comparison with conventional herniorrhaphy. Coala trial group. Annals of Surgery. 1997;**226**:668-675

[23] Swanstron LL. Laparoscopic hernia repairs: The importance of cost as an outcome measurement at the century's end. The Surgical Clinics of North America. 2000;**80**:1341-1351

[24] Bowne WB, Morgenthal CB, Castro AE, et al. The role of endoscopic extraperitoneal herniorrhaphy: Where do we stand in 2005? Surgical Endoscopy. 2007;**21**(5):707-712

[25] Elliott HL, Novitsky YW. Laparascopic inguinal hernia repair. In: Delaney CP, editor. Netter's Surgical Anatomy and Approaches. Philadelphia: Elsevier; 2014. p. 357

[26] Dulucq JL. Tips and Techniques in Laparoscopic Surgery (Totally Extraperitoneal Approach for Laparoscopic Hernia Repair). Berlin: Springer-Verlag; 2005

[27] Kuthe A, Germer CT, Schafmayer A, Tamme C. Standardisierung der TEP Technik. CAMIC Konsensuskonferenz "Leistenhernie". Zentralblatt für Chirurgie. 2003;**128**:586

[28] Lau H, Patil NG, Yuen WK, Lee F. Learning curve for unilateral endoscopic totally extraperitoneal (TEP) inguinal hernioplasty. Surgical Endoscopy. 2002;**16**:1724

[29] Lomanto D, Katara AN. Managing intraoperative complications during totally extraperitoneal repair of inguinal hernia. Journal of Minimal Access Surgery. 2006;**2**:165-170

[30] Simons MP, Aufenacaker T, Bay-Nielsen M, et al. European Hernia Society guidelines on the treatment of inguinal hernia in adult patients. Hernia. 2009;**13**:343-403

[31] Bittner R, Arregui ME, Bisgaard T, et al. Guidelines for laparoscopic (TAPP) and endoscopic (TEP) treatment of inguinal hernia [International EndoHernia Society (IEHS)]. Surgical Endoscopy. 2011;**25**:2773-2843

[32] Welsh DRJ. Sliding inguinal hernias. The Journal of Abdominal Surgery. 1964;**6**:204-209

[33] Dulucq JL, Wintringer P, Mahajna A. Laparoscopic totally extraperitoneal inguinal hernia repair: Lessons learned from 3,100 hernia repairs over 15 years. Surgical Endoscopy. 2009;**23**:482-486

[34] Miguel PR, Reusch M, daRosa AL, Carlos JR. Laparoscopic hernia repair—Complications. JSLS. 1998;**2**:35-40

[35] Ates M et al. Corona mortis: In vivo anatomical knowledge and the risk of injury in totally extraperitoneal inguinal hernia repair. Hernia. 2016;**20**(5):659-665

[36] Kocot A, Gerharz EW, Riedmiller H. Urological complications of laparoscopic inguinal hernia repair: A case series. Hernia. 2011;**15**(5):583-586

[37] Eklund A et al. Chronic pain 5 years after randomized comparison of laparoscopic and Lichtenstein inguinal hernia repair. The British Journal of Surgery. 2010;**97**(4):600-608

[38] Lau H et al. Management of peritoneal tear during endoscopic extra-peritoneal inguinal hernioplasty. Surgical Endoscopy. 2002;**16**(10):1474-1477

[39] Gong K et al. Comparison of the open tension-free mesh-plug, transabdominal preperitoneal (TAPP), and totally extraperitoneal (TEP) laparoscopic techniques for primary unilateral inguinal hernia repair: A prospective randomized controlled trial. Surgical Endoscopy. 2011;**25**(1):234-239

[40] McCormack K et al. Laparoscopic techniques versus open techniques for inguinal hernia repair. Cochrane Database of Systematic Reviews. 2003;**1**:CD001785

Chapter 4

Spigelian Hernia

Bruno Barbosa, Maria João Diogo, César Prudente and Carlos Casimiro

Abstract

Spigelian hernia (SH) is uncommon and accounts for only 0.12–2% of all abdominal hernias. Spigelian hernia is a protrusion through a defect in the aponeurosis of the transversus abdominis muscle (Spigelian fascia) that is limited by the semilunar line and the lateral edge of the rectus abdominis muscle. It is more common in women 50–60 years and it is twice as common on the right side. Patients may present with non-specific abdominal pain. Clinical diagnosis may be difficult, especially in obese patients, and radiologic exams are essential to obtain the correct diagnoses. This type of hernia has a mandatory indication to surgical repair due to the risk of incarceration that can occur in about 25% and strangulation that can occur in about 40%. Traditionally, open surgical repair is most commonly used. However, laparoscopic approach is becoming increasingly popular since it allows faster recovery, shorter hospital stay, and less pain, with no commitment to recurrence. Currently, there are no studies that demonstrate the superiority of a laparoscopic technique (intraperitoneal onlay mesh (IPOM), transabdominal pre-peritoneal (TAPP) or extraperitoneal approach (TEP)). The intraperitoneal route is a simple, faster, and easily reproducible approach.

Keywords: Spigelian hernia, open surgery, intraperitoneal repair laparoscopic surgery, total extraperitoneal repair

1. Introduction

A hernia occurs when there is an abnormal protrusion of an organ or tissue through a natural orifice or weakness point. Abdominal wall hernias are quite frequent, with approximately 700,000 hernia repair surgeries currently performed in the United States every year [1]. There are several types of abdominal wall hernias depending on their location (**Figure 1**), with inguinal hernias being the most common, accounting for 75% of all abdominal wall hernias [1].

Spigelian hernias (SH) are defined as a protrusion of preperitoneal fat, peritoneum or an organ through a defect that can be acquired or congenital, located laterally to the rectus abdominis in the anterior abdominal wall [2, 3]. This type of hernia is rare and has been estimated to account for <2% of all abdominal wall hernias [3–10]. Pain is the most common symptom reported by patients [4, 7], but there are no pathognomonic signs and symptoms, making clinical diagnosis difficult. Complementary diagnostic tests such as ultrasonography (US) and computed tomography (CT) can play an essential role in its diagnosis. Due to the high risk of

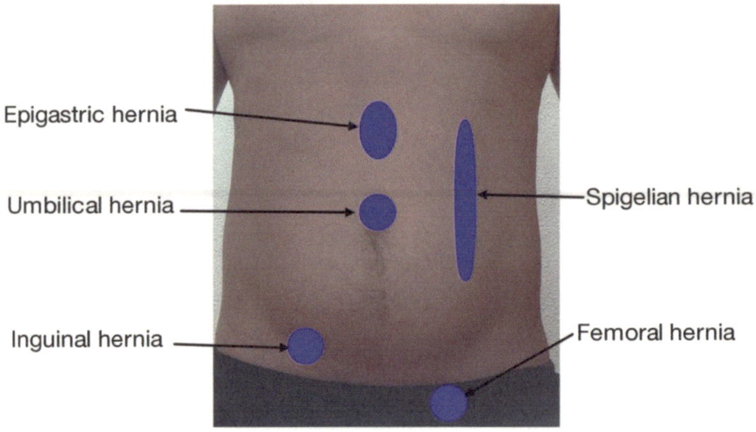

Figure 1.
Different types of abdominal wall hernias.

incarceration (25%) [4, 6, 7], this type of hernia is indicated for surgery [4, 5, 7, 9, 11, 12]. The surgery can be performed openly or laparoscopically, with or without mesh placement [2–18]. Currently, the laparoscopic approach is increasingly used as it is associated with low morbidity rates [2–6, 8, 9, 13, 14]. The laparoscopic approaches described include trans-abdominal approaches such as the intraperitoneal onlay mesh (IPOM), transabdominal pre-peritoneal (TAPP) and totally extra-peritoneal (TEP) techniques [2–5, 9, 11, 14].

2. Anatomy

Spigelian hernia owes its name to the Belgian anatomist Adrian van den Spiegel who first described the semilunar line in 1645 [6–8, 10, 12, 15].

Spiegel described a lateral, convex line extending from the cartilage of the ninth rib to the pubis, lateral to the rectus abdominis and where the transversus abdominis muscle transition to its aponeurosis is found [7, 11]. This line became known as the semilunar line or Spiegel's line (**Figure 2**) [7].

The transversus abdominis muscle aponeurosis that lies between the lateral border of the rectus abdominis muscle medially and the semilunar line laterally is called the Spigelian's fascia or aponeurosis [2, 4–7].

It was not until 1764, more than a century after the description of the semilunar line, that a Spigelian hernia was described for the first time, reported by the Belgian anatomist Josef Klinkosch [3, 6, 8].

This way, SH is defined as a protrusion of preperitoneal fat, peritoneum or an organ through a defect located in the Spigelian fascia [6, 7].

Throughout history, SH has also been called "spontaneous lateral ventral hernia," "semilunar line hernia" and "hernia through the conjoint tendon" [3, 6].

Although SH can occur anywhere on the Spigelian fascia, around 90% occur below the umbilicus, more specifically below the arcuate line [2, 5–8]. This zone is known as the "Spigelian hernia belt" and is defined medially by the lateral border of the rectus abdominis muscle, superiorly by the arcuate line and inferiorly by the inferior epigastric vessels [2–8]. Spigelien's belt is an area about 6 cm wide above a transverse line that passes through the anterior superior iliac spines [5–7].

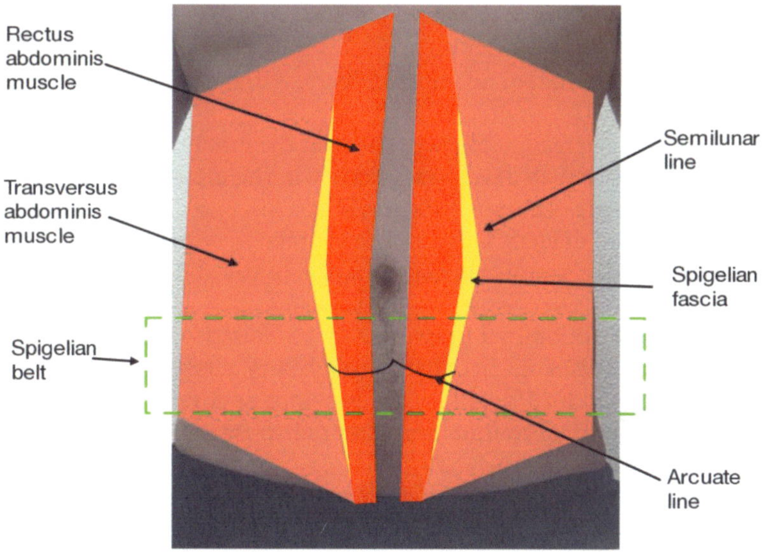

Figure 2.
Anatomy of Spigelian fascia.

The higher incidence of hernias in this location is associated with the fact that in this location the posterior sheath of the rectus abdominis is absent and the fibers of the transversus abdominis and internal oblique muscle are in cross-parallel, making it a weakness point [5–8, 15]. This does not happen above the umbilicus where there is the posterior sheath of the rectus abdominis and the fibers of the transversus abdominis and internal oblique muscles cross perpendicularly [6, 7]. A SH above this area is extremely rare [7].

SH can also occur below and medially to the epigastric vessels and extend to the pubic tubercle, being called "low Spigelian hernia" [7].

The SH sac usually contains extraperitoneal fat, peritoneum, small intestine or omentum, but it may contain other organs such as the stomach, gallbladder, ovaries, testes and bladder [6, 16].

The hernia defect is usually narrow (0.5–2 cm), with rigid margins and covered by the aponeurosis of the external oblique muscle, thus presenting a high risk of incarceration and strangulation [2, 3, 5, 9]. Some studies report that these hernias have a 25% risk of incarceration and 40% of strangulation, making surgical repair a recommendation [4, 6, 7]. Due to the rectus abdominis position, the hernia sac generally expands laterally and caudally along the intraparietal plane between the internal and external oblique muscle [7, 9].

3. Incidence

SH is a rare type of ventral hernia, accounting for about 0.12 to 2% of all hernias [1–3, 6–10, 16]. SH is most commonly diagnosed between age 40 and 70 and is slightly more common in women (male/female ratio 1:1.6) and on the right side of the abdomen (right/left ratio 2:1) [2, 7, 9, 12].

Patients with comorbidities that lead to increased intra-abdominal pressure or weakness of the abdominal wall have the greatest risk of herniation.

4. Pathophysiology and risk factors

SH results from congenital or acquired defects, with a peak incidence in the fifth decade of life [6, 7].

Congenital defects are related to a weak area at the junction of the aponeurosis of the abdominal muscles as they develop separately in the mesenchyme of somatopleure [6, 7]. However, SH rarely occurs in children [7].

Concerning acquired defects, these can be associated with situations that increase intra-abdominal pressure, trauma or degeneration of the abdominal wall aponeurosis [6–8, 15].

The increased intra-abdominal pressure may be caused by situations like chronic obstructive pulmonary disease, chronic cough, obesity, cirrhosis, chronic constipation and pregnancy [6–8, 10, 15]. History of previous abdominal surgery (open or laparoscopic) and abdominal trauma can also predispose to the appearance of SH as it can weaken the semilunar line [6–8, 17].

Some authors have also suggested that the neurovascular opening in Spigelian's aponeurosis may be a susceptible point of herniation; however, this factor is currently considered of little importance [17].

Collagen disorders such as Ehlers-Danlos Syndrome or the aging process can also increase the risk of developing these hernias [6–8].

Therefore, the development of SH is likely to be multifactorial.

5. Clinical presentation

The diagnosis of SH is difficult as there are no characteristic signs or symptoms of this pathology [2, 6, 7, 17].

Unlike other types of hernias, the most common symptom associated with a Spigelian hernia is pain and not a palpable protrusion/mass [2, 4, 5, 7, 17]. SH is often only diagnosed when it becomes symptomatic with incarceration, strangulation or occlusion, and before these events, patients are asymptomatic [7].

Pain varies in type, severity and location depending on the contents of the hernia sac [7, 18]. Typically, the pain is aggravated with standing or any other factor that causes an increase in intra-abdominal pressure, and it improves with rest and with the supine position [3, 7, 18].

In addition to pain, patients may present a palpable mass that may be located far from the hernia orifice [2, 3, 5, 7, 9, 14, 17]. This mass can appear when the patient is standing and disappear spontaneously when lying down [10, 17]. Large SH is easily palpable; however, the diagnosis of hernias with a small hernia sac and orifice is quite challenging [3, 4, 17].

During the physical examination, a tender spot over the hernia defect may be palpated when the abdominal muscles are tense [7, 17]. The sensitivity of the physical examination can be increased by asking the patient to relax and contract the abdomen (Valsalva maneuvers) [7, 18].

The diagnosis is made when a mass and hernia defect is palpated over the Spigelian aponeurosis [3]. However, this clinical presentation is not common since the orifice and hernia sac are rarely detected as it is covered by subcutaneous fat, especially in obese patients, and by the aponeurosis of the external oblique muscle [2–4, 6, 7, 17, 18].

These facts make the clinical diagnosis based only on the physical examination quite difficult, and some studies report that only in 50% of cases, a SH can be detected with only the physical examination [6, 18]. It is therefore essential to complement with diagnostic exams when the patient is in pain but without any palpable mass.

The diagnosis of SH is challenging and requires a high level of suspicion [2–7, 17, 18].

6. Complementary diagnostic exams

As previously mentioned, the diagnosis of SH can be challenging and imaging exams are often necessary to help diagnose or assess the correct diagnosis. These exams are intended to show the presence of a hernia orifice and obtain information about the contents of the hernia sac [3, 4, 8, 14, 17]. Imaging exams also allow us to exclude differential diagnoses, which based only on the clinical presentation can be challenging.

6.1 Abdominal X-ray

In order to be able to make the diagnosis of SH through radiography, the hernia sac must have a subcutaneous location and contain an intestine with air, gas or oral contrast [17]. The use of oral contrast also allows diagnosing occlusion conditions [17]. However, this exam does not allow the diagnosis of SH if the hernia sac contains omentum or if the hernia sac has no content [17]. In these cases, radiography is usually an inconclusive exam [17].

6.2 Ultrasonography (US)

Ultrasonography is recommended as the first-line imaging test to investigate the existence of SH [14, 18], presenting diagnostic utilities on palpable and non-palpable SH [17, 18]. Diagnosis is made when the presence of a hernial orifice in Spigelian aponeurosis is demonstrated [17]. The hernia orifice is visualized as a defect in the echographic line of the aponeurosis (**Figure 3**) [17]. There may also be interruptions in the lines that represent the preperitoneal and peritoneum fat [17]. US has a diagnostic sensitivity of 90% for SH and a positive predictive value of 100% [2]. Thus, US is a highly sensitive and low-cost test, ideal for an initial approach to the diagnosis of SH, but it has the disadvantage of being operator-dependent [15, 18].

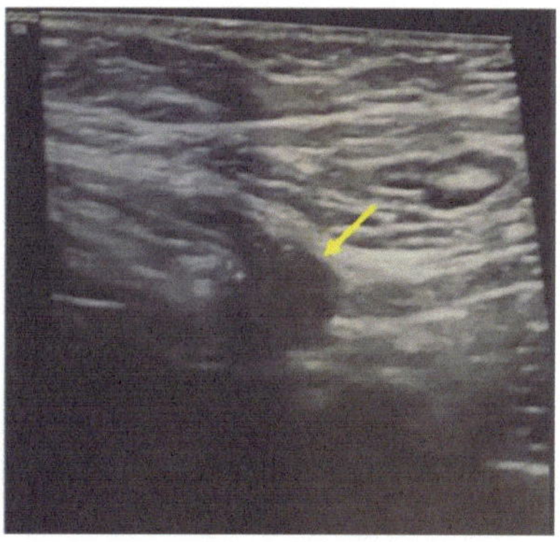

Figure 3.
Ultrasonography of Spigelian hernia (shown by the yellow arrow).

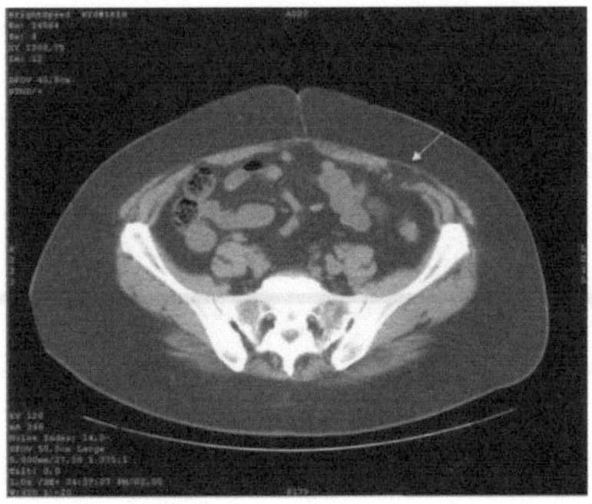

Figure 4.
CT scan of SH orifice (SH shown by the yellow arrow).

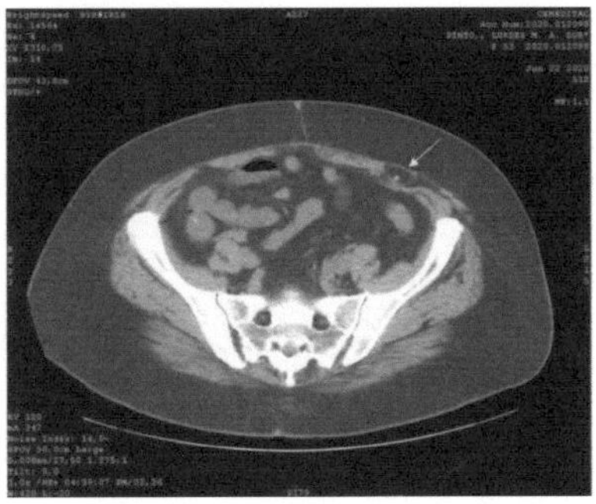

Figure 5.
CT scan of incarcerated SH (SH shown by the yellow arrow).

6.3 Computed tomography (CT)

Some studies suggest that the CT scan has a diagnostic sensitivity of SH of close to 100% [2, 14] and a positive predictive value of 100% [2], making the CT the most reliable exam to perform the diagnosis and delimit the anatomy in uncertain cases (**Figures 4** and **5**) [2, 4, 8, 18].

6.4 Magnetic resonance imaging (MRI)

With the increasing availability, MRI can bring benefits in the preoperative evaluation of doubtful cases [18]. However, more studies are needed to understand its use.

6.5 Laparoscopy

Although US and CT scans are useful tests to make a diagnosis, sometimes SH is not diagnosed by these exams. Thus, when the mass caused by SH is not palpable and is not visible by any imaging exam, exploratory laparoscopy may be indicated [4].

7. Differential diagnosis

SH can have a presentation with several non-specific symptoms, making this pathology easily confused with other intra-abdominal pathologies or lesions of the anterior abdominal wall [7, 17, 18]. The presence of other types of hernias, namely ventral or incisional, the presence of soft tissue or abdominal wall tumors, abscesses or adenopathies should be excluded [7, 17].

Other causes of abdominal pain such as appendicitis, appendicular abscesses and diverticulitis should be excluded [18].

Besides, a hernia can dissect the sheath of the rectus abdominis, making SH to be confused with a spontaneous rupture of the rectum or a hematoma [7].

8. Treatment

As previously mentioned, SH must be treated surgically due to their risk of incarceration and strangulation [2, 4, 7, 9, 11, 17], and up to 1/3 of SH are urgently operated due to these complications [10].

Traditionally, SH was corrected by open surgery; however, with the advances in laparoscopic surgery, it started to play an increasingly important role [2–7]. This approach still allows for a diagnostic acuity of almost 100% [12].

Several studies have shown that laparoscopic surgery has less morbidity, with less pain, fewer operative wound complications and a shorter hospital stay (1–1.4 days vs. 5.2 open days) [2–17].

8.1 Open approach

This procedure is usually performed through a transverse or paramedian incision over the protrusion site [7, 10, 18]. A dissection of the subcutaneous tissue is carried out up to the aponeurosis of the external oblique muscle and its opening with a cut in the direction of the muscle fibers [5, 7, 10, 18, 19]. After reduction of the hernia sac, the hernia orifice can be closed with a non-absorbable suture or with the placement of a synthetic mesh (in a sublay or inlay position) anchored with separate stitches [4, 5, 7, 18, 19].

Some authors advocate that the open route should be chosen if the hernia orifice is larger than 5 cm and if the abdominal wall is visibly damaged [15].

8.2 Laparoscopic approach

In 1992, Carter and Mizes performed the first laparoscopic repair of an SH, having performed a primary suture repair with extracorporeal knotting [5, 11, 12, 14, 18, 19].

The laparoscopic approach allows for an easy location of the defect, requiring less tissue dissection [2, 4, 5, 8, 9, 13]. The use of synthetic mesh is recommended, as it guarantees better results when compared with suture of the hernia defect [4, 11].

Currently, there are three types of laparoscopic approaches with mesh placement described, two through an intra-abdominal approach (IPOM and TAPP) and one through an extraperitoneal approach (TEP). The IPOM approach is the most popular, being performed in about 46.2% of cases, followed by TAPP (35.5%) and TEP (18.3%) [2, 5, 11, 14].

The International Endohernia Society Guidelines Update 2019 recommends that in the laparoscopic treatment of ventral and incisional hernias, an "at least four time the radius of the defect" mesh should be used [4]. Other authors suggest that the mesh should exceed the limits of the hernia defect by 4–5 cm [17, 18].

Laparoscopic approach with the mesh placement is safe, has few complications and allows a faster recovery [2, 5, 11, 12, 14, 15, 17, 18]. However, if we are facing an intra-abdominal infection or signs of strangulation of the contents of the hernia sac, the synthetic mesh should not be used [7].

Given the rarity of this pathology, no study has been able to demonstrate superior outcomes between these three laparoscopic approaches [2, 4–9].

Most studies do not report the existence of SH recurrence after laparoscopic correction regardless of the chosen surgical approach [5, 8, 19].

8.2.1 Intraperitoneal onlay mesh

The IPOM approach is the most commonly used and reported in the literature as it is a technically less demanding approach and fast technique and requires a shorter learning curve compared with others [2, 5, 11, 14]. The IPOM does not require a peritoneal flap and surgeons are more familiar with the intra-abdominal anatomy [5, 14, 17–19].

Brief description of the surgical technique [14, 17, 18]: The patient is positioned supine with both arms along the body. Pneumoperitoneum is performed. Three trocars are introduced: 1 trocar of 10 mm in the mid-clavicular line contralateral to the hernia at the level of the umbilicus or at the umbilicus; 1 trocar of 10 or 5 mm on the midclavicular line in a position superior to the first trocar and the last trocar of 5 mm inferior to the first trocar on the midclavicular line. The content is bluntly reduced and the mesh is placed.

In this technique, a composite or expanded polytetrafluoroethylene (PTFE) mesh is placed to cover the defect, covering at least 5 cm from the circumferential margin of the orifice, and it is anchored with tacks or transabdominal suture [7, 14, 17, 18].

Some studies have shown that intestinal adhesions or erosion of loops can occur due to tacks and the mesh; however, this event has not yet been reported in any clinical case [5, 12, 14]. Another disadvantage of this technique is that it violates the integrity of the abdominal cavity [4, 14].

The IPOM approach has been shown to be safe, with less operative time (mean duration 39 minutes), shorter hospital stay and few complications [5, 14, 17, 18].

8.2.2 Transabdominal preperitoneal approach

The initial approach of TAPP technique is similar to the IPOM [2, 7]; however, unlike the IPOM, the mesh is located anterior to the peritoneum [2, 7, 14, 18]. In this technique, it is necessary to create a peritoneal flap to cover the mesh used making this technique more technically challenging [2, 14, 18]. This flap is then closed with tacks or continuous sutures [18].

As with the IPOM, TAPP also makes it possible to precisely locate the hernia defect and observe the viability of the intestine incarcerated [7, 14, 19].

The TAPP procedure takes an average of 45 minutes [14].

8.2.3 Total extraperitoneal

In 2002 Morena-Egeas described for the first time the correction of SH *via* the TEP technique [13].

Brief description of the surgical technique [2, 5, 7, 10, 11, 18]: Patient in supine position with both arms adducted. Infraumbilical ipsilateral incision and introduction of a 30° optic into a 10-mm port. Creation of a preperitoneal space with carbon dioxide insufflation at a pressure of 10 mmHg or with the inflation of a balloon, followed by telescopic dissection at the midline. Introduction of 2.5-mm working ports in midline, 8 and 3 cm from the pubic symphysis, under a direct view. Dissection and development of a preperitoneal plane. Identification of the hernia sac and mesh placement.

Studies have revealed that patients undergoing correction for TEP require fewer doses of narcotics and less time to resume daily activities when compared with TAPP [11].

TEP has advantages over TAPP since it avoids complications due to the dissection necessary to perform the peritoneal flap and reduces the operative time by avoiding its closure [5, 11, 13]. In addition to these factors, TEP allows the use of a Prolene mesh and does not require the use of tacks to close the peritoneal flap, which reduces the cost of surgery [5, 13]. This technique also makes it possible to reduce possible complications such as iatrogenic lesions of intestine or intestinal obstruction, as there is no violation of the abdominal cavity [5, 11].

However, the disadvantage of TEPP is the inability to do an exploration of the contents of the intestinal sac, making this approach indicated only for elective patients [5, 11].

This approach has an average duration of 59 minutes [14].

TEP is the least used surgical approach as it is the most technically challenging and has a longer learning curve, in addition to requiring a longer hospital stay when compared with IPOM [2, 5].

8.3 Robotic surgery

With the advancement of the availability of robotic surgery, it is expectable that this route of surgical correction will become more and more frequent [7, 20, 21]. SH repair using robotic techniques was described similar to the IPOM laparoscopic approach [7]. Due to the limited number of procedures performed this way, studies have not yet been carried out to determine the effectiveness and safety of robot vs. laparoscopic repairs [20, 21].

A major disadvantage of robotic surgery is the longer surgical time as well as the higher cost [20, 21].

9. Conclusion

Spigelian hernia (SH) is a rare type of abdominal wall hernia and results from protrusion through a defect in the Spigelian aponeurosis. Diagnosis may be difficult, and sometimes, this hernia goes unnoticed on physical examination. It is essential that the physician has a high level of clinical suspicion and often this diagnosis is only possible with the aid of imaging tests (US and CT). This type of hernia has surgical indication due to its risk of incarceration and strangulation. Since it is a rare and underdiagnosed type of hernia, currently there is no surgical technique defined as the ideal one for its correction. The surgical approach chosen must be adjusted to the patient, characteristics of the hernia, the available technical means and the surgeon's experience. Currently, the laparoscopic approach is gradually becoming the preferred surgical approach; however, the open approach remains the most widely used. IPOM approach is the most commonly used, as it is a simple, faster and easily reproducible approach.

Acknowledgements

The authors would like to thank all members of the General Surgery department at Centro Hospitalar Tondela-Viseu for their support and demand for improvement. We highlight the collaboration of Dr. Raquel Pereira, Dr. José Carlos Pereira and Dr. Tiago Pavão.

Conflict of interest

The authors declare no conflict of interest.

Author details

Bruno Barbosa*, Maria João Diogo, César Prudente and Carlos Casimiro
Centro Hospitalar Tondela-Viseu, Viseu, Portugal

*Address all correspondence to: brunobarbosamd@gmail.com

IntechOpen

© 2022 The Author(s). Licensee IntechOpen. This chapter is distributed under the terms of the Creative Commons Attribution License (http://creativecommons.org/licenses/by/3.0), which permits unrestricted use, distribution, and reproduction in any medium, provided the original work is properly cited.

References

[1] Dabbas N, Adams K, Pearson K, Royle G. Frequency of abdominal wall hernias: Is classical teaching out of date? JRSM Short Reports. 2011;**2**(1):5. DOI: 10.1258/shorts.2010.010071

[2] Cui TY, Law TT, Ng L, Wong KY. Spigelian hernia: Our total extraperitoneal approach and a systematic review of the literature. Asian Journal of Endoscopic Surgery. 2021;**14**(3):529-539. DOI: 10.1111/ases.12912

[3] Mederos R, Lamas JR, Alvarado J, Matos M, Padron I, Ramos A. Laparoscopic diagnosis and repair of Spigelian hernia: A case report and literature review. International Journal of Surgery Case Reports. 2017;**31**:184-187. DOI: 10.1016/j.ijscr.2017.01.043

[4] Goulart A, Marques H, Reis M. Hérnia de Spiegel: descrição de caso clínico com análise da literatura. Revista Portuguesa de Cirurgia. 2015;**35**:41-47

[5] Law TT, Ng KK, Ng L, Wong KY. Elective laparoscopic totally extraperitoneal repair for Spigelian hernia: A case series of four patients. Asian Journal of Endoscopic Surgery. 2018;**11**(3):244-247. DOI: 10.1111/ases.12454

[6] Baucom C, Nguyen QD, Hidalgo M, Slakey D. Minimally invasive spigelian hernia repair. JSLS. 2009;**13**(2):263-268

[7] Campanelli G, Pettinari D, Nicolosi FM, Avesani EC. Spigelian hernia. Hernia. 2005;**9**(1):3-5. DOI: 10.1007/s10029-004-0280-z

[8] Yoshida D, Itoh S, Kinjo N, Harimoto N, Maruyama S, Kawanaka H, et al. Laparoscopic intraperitoneal mesh repair of Spigelian hernia: A case report. Asian Journal of Endoscopic Surgery. 2015;**8**(4):477-479. DOI: 10.1111/ases.12205

[9] Filip S, Dragomirescu C, Copăescu C. Laparoscopic treatment of Spiegel hernia by total extraperitoneal (TEP) approach. Chirurgia. 2014;**109**(3):325-329

[10] Kelly ME, Courtney D, McDermott FD, Heeney A, Maguire D, Geoghegan JG, et al. Laparoscopic Spigelian hernia repair: A series of 40 patients. Surgical Laparoscopy, Endoscopy & Percutaneous Techniques. 2015;**25**(3):e86-e89. DOI: 10.1097/SLE.0000000000000112

[11] Donovan K, Denham M, Kuchta K, Carbray J, Ujiki M, Linn J, et al. Laparoscopic totally extraperitoneal and transabdominal preperitoneal approaches are equally effective for spigelian hernia repair. Surgical Endoscopy. 2021;**35**(4):1827-1833. DOI: 10.1007/s00464-020-07582-9

[12] Rankin A, Kostusiak M, Sokker A. Spigelian hernia: Case series and review of the literature. Visceral Medicine. 2019;**35**(2):133-136. DOI: 10.1159/000494280

[13] Moreno-Egea A, Carrasco L, Girela E, Martín JG, Aguayo JL, Canteras M. Open vs laparoscopic repair of spigelian hernia: A prospective randomized trial. Archives of Surgery. 2002;**137**(11):1266-1268. DOI: 10.1001/archsurg.137.11.1266

[14] Dzib-Calan EA, Ortiz-Reyes SF, Morales-Pérez JI, Núñez-Vidales R, Rodarte-Cajica G, Leal-Mérida G. Laparoscopic Spigelian hernia repair with intraperitoneal onlay composite mesh and articulated fixing system. Two cases report. Cirugia y Cirujanos.

2019;**87**(3):353-357. DOI: 10.24875/CIRU.18000484

[15] Ye Z, Wang M-J, Bai L-F, Zhuang H-X, Zhuang W. Spigelian hernia in the right upper abdominal wall: A case report. BMC Surgery. 2018;**18**(1):109. DOI: 10.1186/s12893-018-0449-5

[16] Chaib PS, Coltri RP, de Castro MMO. Hérnia de Spiegel bilateral volumosa. Relatos de Casos. 1900;**0**(4):1-5

[17] Spangen L. Spigelian hernia. World Journal of Surgery. 1989;**13**(5):573-580. DOI: 10.1007/BF01658873

[18] Mittal T, Kumar V, Khullar R, Sharma A, Soni V, Baijal M, et al. Diagnosis and management of Spigelian hernia: A review of literature and our experience. Journal of Minimal Access Surgery. 2008;**4**(4):95-98. DOI: 10.4103/0972-9941.45204

[19] Barnes TG, McWhinnie DL. Laparoscopic Spigelian hernia repair: A systematic review. Surgical Laparoscopy, Endoscopy & Percutaneous Techniques. 2016;**26**(4):265-270. DOI: 10.1097/SLE.0000000000000286

[20] Jamshidian M, Stanek S, Sferra J, Jamil T. Robotic repair of symptomatic Spigelian hernias: A series of three cases and surgical technique review. Journal of Robotic Surgery. 2018;**12**(3):557-560. DOI: 10.1007/s11701-017-0742-9

[21] Gonzalez A, Escobar E, Romero R, Walker G, Mejias J, Gallas M, et al. Robotic-assisted ventral hernia repair: A multicenter evaluation of clinical outcomes. Surgical Endoscopy. 2017;**31**(3):1342-1349. DOI: 10.1007/s00464-016-5118-0

Chapter 5

Spigelian Hernia: Clinical Features and Management

Aakansha Giri Goswami, Farhanul Huda, Sudhir Kumar Singh, Navin Kumar and Somprakas Basu

Abstract

The Spigelian hernia is a rare variety of ventral hernia and has an incidence ranging from 0.1–2% of all abdominal wall hernias. It occurs through a well-defined defect in the Spiegel's fascia adjacent to the semilunar line. It can be congenital or acquired. The acquired variety is predisposed by stretching and weakening of the abdominal wall by factors that increase the intraabdominal pressure. These hernias are most commonly located in the interparietal plane with no visible or palpable mass, and only 50% of cases could be diagnosed clinically before any surgical intervention. Radiological investigations like USG and CT scans confirm the clinical diagnosis or pick up the subclinical varieties that present with non-specific pain in the anterior abdominal wall. Surgery is the mainstay of management. These hernias are prone to early incarceration and strangulation and therefore should be operated at the earliest. It is stressed that a prosthetic mesh should be used for a better outcome as it decreases recurrence. Conventional open hernioplasty has been largely replaced by a laparoscopic approach such as TAPP, TEP, IPOM and robotic-assisted surgery. Early diagnosis and surgery prevent morbidity and dreaded complications.

Keywords: hernia, abdominal hernia, ventral hernia, Spigelian hernia, Spigelian fascia

1. Introduction

Hernias penetrating the anterior abdominal wall are considered the ventral hernias, and the majority of these are formed by the inguinal, femoral and umbilical hernia. Rare varieties include the lumbar and Spigelian hernias. The Spigelian hernias, principally acquired, has an incidence ranging from 0.1–2% of all abdominal wall hernias [1, 2]. These hernias occur through a well-defined defect in the Spiegel's fascia of the anterior abdominal wall adjacent to the semilunar line, which corresponds anatomically to the lateral edge of the rectus abdominis muscle. These hernias, therefore, are also known as the "spontaneous lateral ventral hernia" or "hernia of the semilunar line". Commonly it occurs at the lower part of the abdomen, below the umbilicus where the posterior rectus sheath is deficient.

2. History

The semilunar line, originally named the "linea semilunaris spigelii" (the line of Spiegel), is named after the Flemish anatomist and surgeon, Adrian van der Spiegel (1578–1625) who first described the anatomical and surgical significance of well-known linea semilunaris [1]. He defined it as the line of transition between the muscle and aponeurosis of transversus abdominis muscle, extending from the ninth costal cartilage to the pubic tubercle with a lateral convexity sometimes easily described as the lateral border of the rectus sheath. Although, Spiegel first described the linea semilunaris, it was not until more than hundred years later the Spigelian hernia was first described clinically by another Flemish anatomist and surgeon Josef Thaddaei Klinkosh in the year 1764, setting forth the surgical significance of this line [3]. He described it as a ventral hernia developing at the site of linea spigelii, and distinctively coined the name Spigelian hernia.

3. Surgical anatomy

The Spigelian line marks the transition from transverse abdominis muscle to aponeurosis. The part of this aponeurosis that lies lateral to the rectus abdominis muscle is called Spigelian fascia/aponeurosis. Hence Spigelian aponeurosis is limited medially by the lateral edge of the rectus muscle and laterally by the semilunar line. Thus, anatomically the Spigelian fascia is the medial part of the transversus aponeurosis between the lateral border of the rectus sheath and semilunar line and stretches from the tip of the 9th costal cartilage until the pubic tubercle. The Spigelian hernia can occur at any point through this fascia.

The crescentic shape and wide variability in the width of Spigelian aponeurosis craniocaudally predispose to the specific site of these hernia formations (**Figure 1**). The Spigelian line in the cranial part of the abdominal wall lies close to the rectus abdominis muscle, and hence the Spigelian aponeurosis is very narrow in this zone, due to the presence of more muscular three flat muscles of the abdominal wall attaching to the lateral border of the rectus sheath. Thereby the muscular fibres and aponeurosis of the external and internal oblique muscles overlap the narrow Spigelian aponeurosis. This is probably the main reason why these hernias are uncommonly

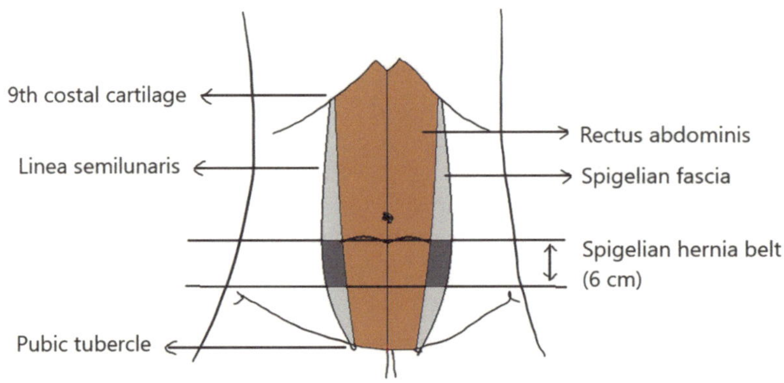

Figure 1.
Schematic diagram showing the Spigelian fascia and Spigelian hernia belt.

found above the umbilicus. It is also seen that the fibres of the internal oblique and transverse abdominis muscle run at an angle to each other above the umbilicus thereby providing additional strength and preventing hernia formation. More commonly these hernias are located in an approximately 6 cm transverse imaginary zone extending from the interspinal line to 6 cm superior to it. The Spigelian fascia is widest here with the greatest abdominal circumference and highest intra-abdominal pressure. Due to its etiological significance, this belt is aptly known as the Spigelian hernia belt [4].

The size of the hernia orifices usually ranges from 0.5 to 2 cm in diameter. It has a well-defined, firm edge and is round to oval in shape (**Figure 2**). This well-defined, fibrous, inelastic edge is believed to increase the risk of incarceration and leads to a condition akin to Richter's hernia formation [5–9]. In the beginning, these hernias are usually limited to the Spigelian aponeurosis on the axial plane, but when their size increases, these can dissect the fibres of transverse abdominis muscles laterally as its medial extension is limited by the rectus muscle and sheath, and create a bigger defect in the anterior abdominal wall. Another probable reason for its lateral position is because that the external oblique aponeurosis covers the Spigelian aponeurosis in its whole length and creates a potential space between the muscle layers. This provides enough space for the herniated sac to expand and take the route of least resistance laterally and is thus palpable more lateral than the actual location of the hernia orifice. This usually conforms to a mushroom-shaped appearance of these hernias on palpation.

In most patients, due to the presence of the tough external oblique aponeurosis, a small Spigelian hernia may go unnoticed. For the Spigelian hernia to be palpable clinically, it needs to penetrate both the transverse abdominis, internal oblique muscles and further glide in between the two oblique muscles. Further, the dissection of the internal oblique is determined by the fact whether the internal oblique muscle ventral to Spigelian aponeurosis is aponeurotic or muscular. In the event the hernial sac encounters an aponeurotic layer in its way, the hernia sac will tend to lie between the transversus abdominis and the internal oblique muscles. Although, the aponeurosis of the internal oblique muscle strengthens the Spigelian fascia, more often than not it is the internal oblique muscle belly rather than the aponeurosis that covers the Spigelian

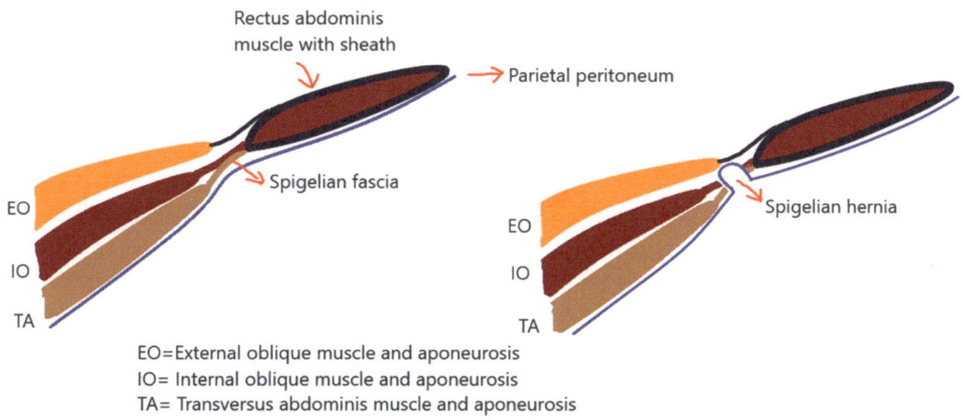

Figure 2.
Schematic diagram showing herniation through the Spigelian hernia. Note the hernial sac is obscured under the external oblique aponeurosis.

fascia, thereby reducing the reinforcement. In cases when the hernial sac grows and dissects the two innermost muscle layers, the hernia may become palpable clinically. Most commonly these are palpable below the level of the umbilicus as the fibres of the transversus abdominis and internal oblique muscles run parallel to each other in this area, thus reducing the resistance further. Above the umbilicus, these muscle fibres form a criss-cross configuration providing additional support and resistance and thereby decreasing the chance of a Spigelian hernia to be palpable but at the same time increasing the chance for incarceration.

It was usually believed that Spigelian hernias tend to occur through small defects in the transversus abdominis aponeurosis where it was penetrated by the perforating vessels and nerves [10, 11]. These were also thought to occur at the junction of the semilunar line and semicircular line of Douglas as the majority of cases were described below the umbilicus in the region of the line of Douglas. This observation was attributed to the fact that not only Spigelian fascia is broadest here but also the lack of posterior rectus sheath represents the inherent weakness of this zone, and also due to fibres of transversus aponeurosis that runs parallel to the internal oblique. This concept was first challenged by Webber et al., who demonstrated that approximately 45% of Spigelian hernias occurred above the arcuate line [12]. Interestingly, although most of these hernias can occur in the Spigelian hernia belt below the umbilicus for the aforementioned reasons [13, 14], the defect may still lie above the arcuate line. The hernia sac usually consists of the peritoneum, preperitoneal fat and occasionally transversalis fascia. The hernial content can be small bowel or omentum but can include any organ depending on its location. The size of the neck has been reported to vary from as small as 0.5 cm to as large as 6 cm [15].

4. Pathophysiology

These hernias can be congenital or acquired. Congenital cases develop through the weak areas in the aponeurosis of the abdominal muscles formed during their development in the mesenchyme of the somatopleure originating from the invading and fusing myotomes of the anterior abdominal wall and are usually associated with cryptorchidism [14, 16]. The congenital variety presents in the younger age, is usually small and mostly remains subclinical. Adult hernias are usually acquired. The perforating vessels were believed to create the area of weakness in the Spigelian fascia which was enhanced by herniation of preperitoneal fat, although this is now considered of minor importance [17]. Spigelian fascia is widest below the umbilicus and potentially weakest. Besides, the abdominal girth is wider below the umbilicus and in accordance with the Laplace's law, wall tension will be greater. Furthermore, transversus abdominis and internal oblique muscles in the upper part of the abdomen extent medially into the posterior rectus sheath and strengths the Spigelian fascia. The natural progression of the disease ranges from younger patients usually presenting with a smaller fascial defect with preperitoneal tissue being the most common content. However, with increasing age, elderlies are vulnerable to the development of larger defects with peritoneal contents constituting the main sac content [18].

Besides the anatomical factors, hernia formation can be predisposed by stretching of the abdominal wall by factors that increase the intraabdominal pressure such as chronic cough, chronic obstructive pulmonary disease, obesity, ascites, pregnancy. It has also been described as a complication of chronic ambulatory peritoneal dialysis [19, 20].

Besides these, scarring from previous abdominal surgeries, paralysis of the anterior abdominal wall may weaken the Spigelian aponeurosis and create an area of weakness [21].

It has also been reported that the creation of pneumoperitoneum during laparoscopic surgeries can predispose to herniation through a pre-existing weakness in the Spigelian fascia [22].

5. Epidemiology

The true prevalence of Spigelian hernia remains elusive as the majority of these cases are asymptomatic. A recent study showed that on ultrasonographic examination of 785 anterior abdominal wall hernias, only 1.4% of patients had Spigelian hernias indicating the rarity of the condition [23]. In another study, 2% of incidental Spigelian defect was identified during laparoscopic procedure further affirming the uniqueness of this hernia [24]. Spigelian hernias are slightly more common in females, occur mostly on the right side and usually affect people in their fourth to the seventh decades of life [25–27]. However, the laterality of these hernias is a contentious issue and as in other studies, left side location has shown predominance [28, 29]. Nevertheless, the underlying reasons are unknown and laterality remains inconsequential to its management.

6. Clinical features

The majority of these hernias are asymptomatic and accordingly the diagnosis is difficult, especially when these are of smaller size. The intraparietal location with overlying tough external oblique aponeurosis and thick subcutaneous fat mask their detection during a clinical examination. However, in patients who present with symptoms, these may range from nonspecific abdominal pain to a palpable lump or a visible mass in the abdominal wall to dangerous features of incarceration with or without features of strangulation. The characteristic of pain depends on the size and contents of the hernia. This may be a dull, sharp, or even burning type. However, one symptom is usually constant, and the pain is aggravated with increased intraabdominal pressure and often after a heavy meal, exercise, walking and running, and is relieved with rest and lying down. Nonetheless, the occult nature of these hernias predisposes them to incarceration and the risk of strangulation requiring emergency laparotomy is up to 24% [30–32] which is way above the 5-year strangulation risk of umbilical hernia (4%) and inguinal hernia (2.5%) [33, 34].

In cases of a visible lump, it is delineated when the anterior abdominal wall is made taut and the patient is in the upright position, but disappears when the patient lies down. With the increase in size, the lump tends to expand laterally and caudally between the layers of two oblique muscles. Therefore, at times, the patient may present with a non-specific bulge without a definite well-demarcated palpable lump which may be due to a typical T-shaped hernial sac causing elevation of the intact external oblique aponeurosis. The diagnosis of hernia can be affirmed if the swelling can be reduced, but reappears in the upright position and especially with the manoeuvres that increase intraabdominal pressure such as coughing, straining or a Valsalva manoeuvre, and disappears on lying down.

Palpation of the hernia defect in most cases is difficult as these defects are small and are masked by the tough external oblique aponeurosis and subcutaneous fat. However, an attempt should be made to palpate the abdominal wall after making the musculature taut to identify any local tenderness indicating the point of the hernial orifice, which may be the only sign in case of occult or a subclinical Spigelian hernia. This may be attributed to the fact that reinforcing manoeuvres that increase intraabdominal pressure pushes out the preperitoneal fat or a hernial sac through the defect. Palpation of these structures against the inelastic margin of the hernial orifice and stimulation of stretch receptors located in the parietal peritoneum produce distinct point tenderness which is more of somatic pain in nature and hence is easily localised [35]. Although, not pathognomonic, this examination has high sensitivity and can help in screening patients with occult herniation. Sometimes, patients report extreme tactile hyperesthesia which is located just medial to the hernia defect. This is generally believed to be caused by mechanical irritation of the perforating branch of the corresponding intercostal nerve (Valleix phenomena) and this sign can aid in clinical diagnosis of a subclinical herniation [36]. For patients presenting with abdominal pain but no visible lump, radiological investigations like ultrasonogram and/or CT-scan of the abdomen can be of foremost importance. Furthermore, in cases where the diagnosis remains elusive even after radiological investigations, a diagnostic laparoscopy may be of help [28].

7. Diagnosis

These hernias are most commonly located in the interparietal plane with no visible or palpable mass as discussed above, and only 50% of cases could be diagnosed clinically before any surgical intervention [17]. Their tendency to masquerade other clinical conditions presenting with abdominal pain requires a high index of clinical suspicion.

The most common symptoms are mild pain aggravated by coughing, straining, exercising and being relieved by lying down. Although, occasionally a lump may be noted, the diagnosis is often missed unless the patient presents with partial bowel obstruction. The clinical examination alone is believed to be 100% sensitive with a PPV of 36% when compared with operative findings [35].

The diagnostic imaging mainly aims at identifying the hernia defect, sac and its content.

7.1 X-rays

It is a poor modality for diagnosing these hernias. It can neither aid in demonstrating the defect nor the content, especially the omentum or preperitoneal fat. However, in cases in which the sac contains a portion of the small or large bowel, barium studies can be of help. Besides, for diagnosing the complications of these hernias such as intestinal obstruction, a conventional x-ray can be used.

7.2 Ultrasonography (USG)

It is considered the investigation of choice and is usually the first-line imaging modality often used. It should be performed in patients presenting with obscure pain in the abdomen with or without a lump and is helpful both in clinical and subclinical hernias. It helps in the identification of a hernia defect, sac, and its content. It has the additional advantage of providing real-time scanning images by changing the patient's position and performing manoeuvres that increase the intraabdominal pressure and precipitates any fascial defects or herniation of fat or viscus.

Using a 3.5 MHz transducer, the examination is first performed with the patient in the supine position and the abdominal wall relaxed. A screening USG is performed for intraabdominal viscera to rule out any potential intraabdominal pathology as a cause of pain. Next a higher denomination transducer, typically 5 MHz is used for the parietal wall structures. Scanning is begun at the lateral end of the rectus muscle with parasagittal sweeps. This helps in visualising the rectus muscle. In longitudinal scans, echogenic strips can be visualised, the deepest of which is the parietal layer, more superficial are the layers of the ventral wall. The hernia defect is seen as a disruption of these echogenic strips (**Figure 3**). The visualisation of the defect and the interparietal location of the sac represent the typical Spigelian hernia with omentum as its content. In difficult cases, the patient may be instructed to increase intraabdominal pressure through Valsalva manoeuvre, which may demonstrate the fascial disruption, and herniation of preperitoneal fat or abdominal viscus. In correlation with the operative findings, a real-time USG scan is believed to have a sensitivity of 90% and PPV of 100% [35].

7.3 Computed Tomography (CT) scan

It is considered as effective as the USG for demonstration of the hernial orifice. Additionally, it provides better information of abdominal wall resistance. Overall,

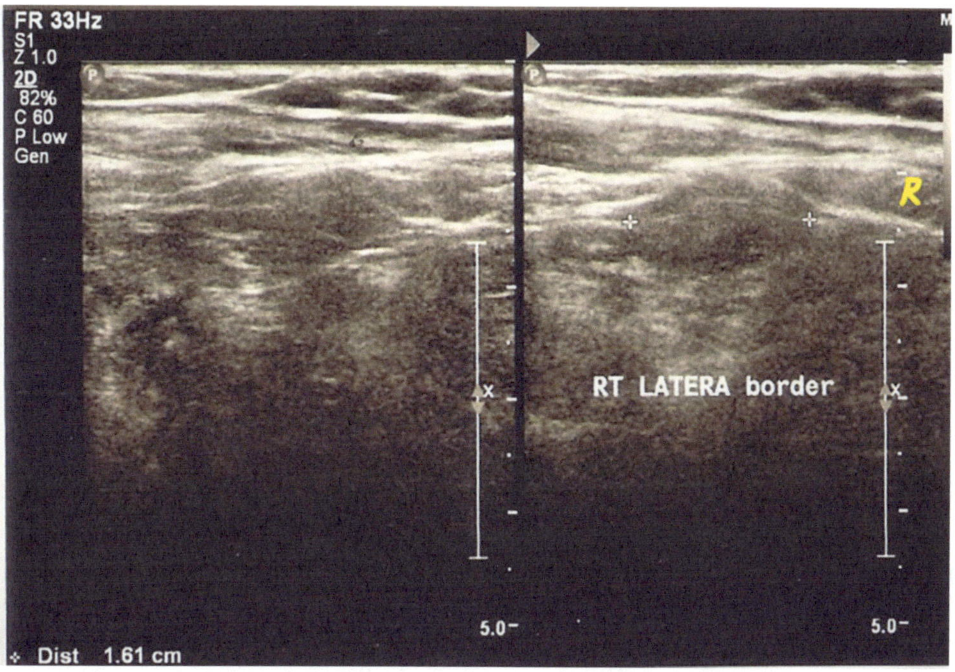

Figure 3.
Dynamic USG of the abdominal wall showing a Spigelian hernial sac (1.6 cm) penetrating through the Spigelian fascia, seen here as a broken line in the muscle-fascial plane. The right rectus muscle is marked as "R" in yellow.

the CT scan has a sensitivity and PPV of 100% each when compared with operative findings [35]. But, the USG is easier to perform, is a clinic procedure, is less expensive and can help in the dynamic analysis of the patient for which it is an excellent screening tool for the lesion. In cases where USG gives inadequate or equivocal information, a CT scan should be added.

7.4 Surgical exploration

On many occasions, the preoperative diagnosis may remain obscure until surgical exploration is performed. In a study by Weiss et al., approximately 50 percent of cases are diagnosed on exploration [37].

Therefore, for diagnosing Spigelian hernias, a dynamic USG and CT scan are useful when used in tandem with the clinical examination. In cases of uncertainty, diagnostic laparoscopy can be used in a symptomatic patient.

8. Differential diagnosis

Depending on its location, a Spigelian hernia may mimic intra-abdominal pathologies which can present with pain such as acute appendicitis, twisted ovarian cyst, tubo-ovarian pathologies, mesenteric lymphadenitis, biliary colic, peptic ulcer pain, pancreatic pain or mesenteric ischemia [35]. Many times one may confuse it with any other disease entity of the abdominal parietal wall too. If the hernia is palpable at the location of pain and if it is reducible, the diagnosis is easy. In instances when the lump is palpable in a typical location but not reducible, the differential diagnoses include hematoma of rectus abdominis muscle, lipoma, chronic abscess, lymphadenopathy, other ventral hernias, solid tumours of the abdominal wall such as a desmoid tumour [35]. In cases where it is not palpable and the patient presents with non-specific pain or if a mass is present in the ventral wall, which is irreducible, the first step is directed towards identifying the nature of the swelling by a dynamic USG. If a Spigelian hernia is suspected, the attempt should be made to localise the hernial orifice. USG can help in differentiating hematoma, abscess, lipoma or seroma. Myotendinitis of rectus abdominis or external oblique muscle can mimic the tenderness present in subclinical cases. In cases where the defect is not found, and diagnosis is obscured, patients should be worked up and investigated for gastrointestinal and genitourinary disorders. An abdominal CT scan reinforces the diagnosis or helps in excluding the differential diagnoses, particularly whether the pain arises from the intra-abdominal pathologies or from the parietal abdominal wall. It is important to keep in mind that in a difficult clinical situation where the diagnosis is elusive or when a subclinical Spigelian hernia is suspected, every effort should be made to rule out an intra-abdominal pathology first. In the pursuit of diagnosing a suspected Spigelian hernia, an important intra-abdominal pathology should not be missed.

9. Classification

Spigelian hernias are the subgroup of primary ventral hernias and the European Hernia Society (EHS) classification system is most commonly used for their classification [38]. However, Webber et al. (2017) have described three clinical stages which reflect the natural history of the condition and provide universality for their management (**Table 1**) [12].

Stages	Anatomy	Clinical Feature	Treatment
I	Defect: <2 cm Content: interstitial fat only with no peritoneal component	Intermittent, well-localised pain but no palpable swelling	Open surgery: they are not visible laparoscopically
II	Defect: 2–5 cm Content: peritoneal component present	Palpable swelling	Laparoscopy/Open repair
III	Defect: >5 cm	Large hernia with distortion the of abdominal wall	Open repair

Table 1.
Clinical stages of Spigelian hernia.

10. Treatment

Operative management of these hernias is advisable as the risk of strangulation or incarceration has been reported up to 25% [39]. Initially open anterior approach with primary closure of the defect or mesh placement in cases where primary closure was not possible was advised. With the technical progress of laparoscopy, its use in the diagnosis and repair of Spigelian hernias has made it the method of choice [40]. It provides the benefits of minimally invasive surgery like reduced post-operative pain, less chance of infection, shorter hospital stays, reduction in morbidity and better cosmesis. However, according to the recent EHS guidelines, it is suggested that Spigelian hernia should be repaired with mesh. The approach, either open or laparoscopic may depend on the surgeon's expertise, because the strength of recommendation is weak as limited comparative data is available [41]. A randomised trial comparing 11 conventional and 11 laparoscopic repairs in elective Spigelian hernia surgery revealed significant advantages for laparoscopic repair in terms of morbidity (wound complications) and hospital stay [42].

The most popular laparoscopic repairs are the Intraperitoneal Onlay Mesh (IPOM) technique (35%), Total Extraperitoneal Patch (TEP) approach (30%), Transabdominal Preperitoneal (TAPP) approach (22%), and laparoscopic suturing techniques [43, 44]. The TEP repair of Spigelian hernia offers the advantage of avoiding breach in the peritoneal layer as it accesses only through the preperitoneal space. Although, studies have failed to demonstrate the superiority of the extraperitoneal approach over intraperitoneal repair, the intraperitoneal laparoscopic Spigelian hernia repair is considered the gold standard because of its technical advantages [45].

11. Operative techniques

11.1 Conventional open approach

A transverse incision is placed over the lump and the external oblique is incised in its direction to expose the peritoneal sac which can simply be inverted (**Figure 4**). The hernia defect can be closed with sutures but in cases of larger defect, a mesh should be used which is placed either in preperitoneal space or above the fascia.

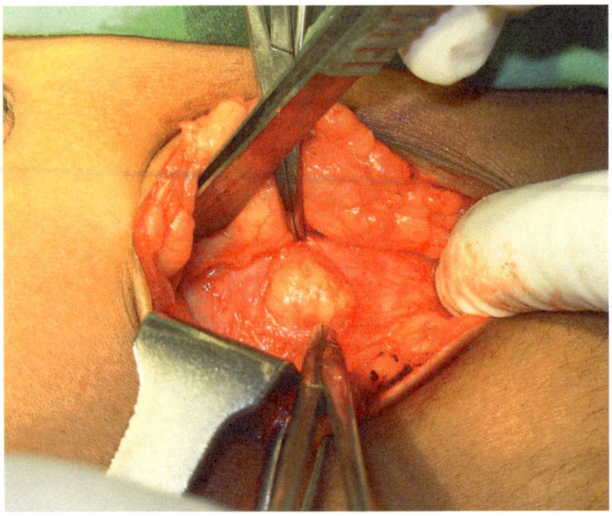

Figure 4.
Open surgical repair of a subclinical Spigelian hernia containing protrusion of preperitoneal fat only (sacless).

11.2 Laparoscopic transabdominal preperitoneal repair (TAPP)

Once the hernial sac contents are reduced, the preperitoneal flap is raised and dissected for 5 cm around the hernial defect. The mesh is placed in the extraperitoneal space and the peritoneal flap is closed. The TAPP provides the opportunity to explore the abdominal cavity, although a potential drawback may be the possibility of intraperitoneal adhesions after the surgery, the chances of which, however, are almost similar to that of other laparoscopic surgery. At times, difficulty in the closure of the peritoneal flap may be encountered because of the thin and fragile peritoneum in this location [45].

11.3 Laparoscopic total extraperitoneal repair (TEP)

The extraperitoneal space is created by open access and a balloon is used to create and enlarge the working space. The hernial sac is identified and closed. A large mesh is used to cover the hernia defect and is fixed to the abdominal wall. Although, this approach prevents access to the intraperitoneal cavity for inspection of any concomitant pathology, it reduces the risk of adhesions [46] besides possible benefit to explore and treat the concomitant direct inguinal hernia [47]. TEP repair is expensive due to the price of balloon dissector, technically challenging with a longer learning curve [48] and can be used only if the hernia is located below the arcuate line [49].

11.4 Intraperitoneal onlay mesh repair (IPOM)

Intraperitoneal access is gained using either closed or open techniques. The hernial site is identified and port placement is done in the form of an arc or a circle with the centre at the defect site which should be at least 10 cm away. The contents are reduced and a coated mesh is fixed to obtain an overlap of at least 5 cm around the defect. It provides the opportunity to explore the abdominal cavity and therefore is helpful in emergency conditions with the incarcerated hernia [50, 51]. It is also believed to be the easiest to learn and safe to perform [52]. Nonetheless, the main limitation to this technique is the risk of hematoma formation and nerve entrapment after tack or stapler application. The use of fibrin sealant in place of tacks provides the solution [53].

11.5 Robotic-assisted technique

The use of robotics on ventral wall hernias are easier due to a 360-degree rotation, camera use, surgical forceps and excellent visualisation of the defect. The placement of sutures also makes the procedure easier. The postoperative pain score reported is also lower [54]. Although, robotic-assisted Spigelian hernia surgery provides technical advantage and reliability, further studies with longer follow-ups are required for conclusive analysis [55].

Postoperative complications include seroma and hematoma formation, surgical site infection, abdominal viscera injury, mesh infection, and recurrence. Nerve entrapment during mesh-tacker placement can lead to abdominal pain syndromes [55].

12. Low Spigelian hernias

Spigelian aponeurosis extends caudally up to the pubic tubercle and is found medial to the inferior epigastric artery within the Hasselbach's triangle. Hernias penetrating the fascia transversalis here are conveniently called the low Spigelian hernias. These hernias usually contain preperitoneal fat but occasionally the bladder may also be involved.

Direct inguinal hernias are located at a similar triangle and may therefore cause diagnostic confusion. Differentiating these hernias from the direct inguinal hernia is important because the risk of incarceration is higher. Due to a small but well-defined hernia orifice, hernioplasty is easier to perform with a lesser chance of recurrence. Digital palpation with the little finger in the inguinal canal in standing position and Valsalva manoeuvre touches the first phalanx in case of low Spigelian hernia and the middle one in direct inguinal hernia. This technique has been proposed to distinguish between these two hernias, but can be uncomfortable and even painful for the patient. The diagnosis can be confirmed by radiological investigation and final assessment is best done intraoperatively [56]. Although, very rare, if both the hernias are found it is most likely due to weakness of Spigelian fascia around the insertion of rectus abdominis [45].

13. Subclinical Spigelian hernia: the great masquerader

The diagnosis of a small Spigelian hernia is extremely challenging, given its rarity combined with nonspecific pain symptoms. Secondly, often due to its intramural location, its detection by palpation can be extremely difficult. Therefore, a great deal of clinical intelligence is invested in its preoperative diagnosis and the ignorance of its existence can cumulate to catastrophic complications of strangulation. Often only a point tenderness corresponding to the site of the defect is the only finding on palpation of the abdominal wall after making the muscles taut [57]. These hernias are small and often may contain only the preperitoneal fat protrusion through the fascial defect (**Figure 4**), which is something similar to the sacless epigastric hernia. As mentioned previously, only less than half of the cases are detected preoperatively. Therefore, patients presenting with non-specific pain in the abdomen should alert the astute clinician for the possibility of a Spigelian hernia. Once the diagnosis is established, treatment is elementary with surgery being the treatment of choice in symptomatic cases.

14. Conclusion

Spigelian hernias are notoriously difficult to diagnose. If these are visible and palpable, diagnosis is straight forward. But if the hernia is subclinical, it is difficult to diagnose, and only radiological investigations such as a dynamic USG or CT-scan of the abdomen wall can pick up the lesion. A strong clinical suspicion helps to diagnose the occult variety, which presents as non-specific abdominal pain, otherwise about 50% remain undiagnosed until surgery. Due to the high risk of incarceration and strangulation, these hernias should be operated early. Open conventional surgery has been largely replaced by laparoscopic mesh hernioplasty.

Funding

Nil.

Conflict of interest

Authors declare no conflict of interest.

Author details

Aakansha Giri Goswami, Farhanul Huda, Sudhir Kumar Singh, Navin Kumar and Somprakas Basu*
Department of General Surgery, All India Institute of Medical Sciences, Rishikesh, India

*Address all correspondence to: somprakas.surg@aiimsrishikesh.edu.in

IntechOpen

© 2022 The Author(s). Licensee IntechOpen. This chapter is distributed under the terms of the Creative Commons Attribution License (http://creativecommons.org/licenses/by/3.0), which permits unrestricted use, distribution, and reproduction in any medium, provided the original work is properly cited.

References

[1] Houlihan TJ. A review of spigelian hernias. American Journal of Surgery. 1976;**131**(6):734-735

[2] Leon SJ, Acevedo EA, Dellepiane PV. Hernia de Spiegel. Revista Chilena de Cirugía. 2011;**63**(1):64-68

[3] Klinkosch JT. Programma quo divisionem herniarum, novamque herniae ventralis speciem proponit. Pragae, Clauser; 1764

[4] Spangen L. Spigelian hernia. Acta Chirurgica Scandinavica. Supplementum. 1976;**462**:1-47

[5] River LP. Spigelian hernia: Spontaneous lateral ventral hernia through the semilunar line. Annals of Surgery. 1942;**116**(3):405-411

[6] Balthazar EJ, Subramanyam BR, Megibow A. Spigelian hernia: CT and ultrasonography diagnosis. Gastrointestinal Radiology. 1984; **9**(1):81-84

[7] Naylor J. Combination of Spigelian and Richter's hernias: A case report. The American Surgeon. 1978;**44**(11):750-752

[8] Som PM, Khilnani MT, Wolf BS, Beranbaum SL. Spigelian hernia. Acta Radiologica: Diagnosis (Stockh). 1976; **17**(3):305-312

[9] Sheehan V. Spigelian hernia. Journal of the Irish Medical Association. 1951;**29**(172):87-91

[10] London P. The anatomy and surgical treatment of inguinal and congenital hernia. The Edinburgh Medical and Surgical Journal. 1806;**2**(6):241-251

[11] Robinson HB. A clinical lecture on hernia through the semilunar line and direct inguinal hernia: Delivered at St. Thomas's hospital, London. British Medical Journal. 1908;**2**(2490):781-782. DOI: 10.1136/bmj.2.2490.781

[12] Webber V, Low C, Skipworth RJE, Kumar S, de Beaux AC, Tulloh B. Contemporary thoughts on the management of Spigelian hernia. Hernia. 2017;**21**(3):355-361

[13] Polistina FA, Garbo G, Trevisan P, Frego M. Twelve years of experience treating Spigelian hernia. Surgery. 2015;**157**(3):547-550

[14] Skandalakis PN, Zoras O, Skandalakis JE, Mirilas P. Spigelian hernia: Surgical anatomy, embryology, and technique of repair. The American Surgeon. 2006;**72**(1):42-48

[15] Lawler MR Jr, Carlisle BB. Giant spigelian hernia. American Journal of Surgery. 1966;**111**(4):562-564

[16] Jones BC, Hutson JM. The syndrome of Spigelian hernia and cryptorchidism: A review of paediatric literature. Journal of Pediatric Surgery. 2015;**50**(2):325-330

[17] Olson RO, Davis WC. Spigelian hernia: Rare or obscure? American Journal of Surgery. 1968;**116**(6): 842-846

[18] Huttinger R, Sugumar K, Baltazar-Ford KS. Spigelian Hernia. StatPearls [Internet]. Treasure Island (FL): StatPearls Publishing; 2022

[19] Malazgirt Z, Topgul K, Sokmen S, Ersin S, Turkcapar AG, Gok H, et al. Spigelian hernias: A prospective analysis of baseline parameters and surgical outcome of 34 consecutive patients. Hernia. 2006;**10**(4):326-330

[20] Engeset J, Youngson GG. Ambulatory peritoneal dialysis and hernial complications. The Surgical Clinics of North America. 1984;**64**(2):385-392

[21] Beyer U. On hernias of the linea semilunaris (Spigelii). Zentralblatt für Chirurgie. 1967;**92**(33):2373-2376

[22] Slakey DR, Teplitsky S, Cheng SS. Incarcerated Spigelian hernia following laparoscopic living-donor nephrectomy. JSLS: Journal of the Society of Laparoendoscopic Surgeons. 2002;**6**(3):217-219

[23] Smereczyński A, Kołaczyk K, Lubiński J, Bojko S, Gałdyńska M, Bernatowicz E. Sonographic imaging of Spigelian hernias. Journal of Ultrasonography. 2012;**12**(50):269-275

[24] Paajanen H, Ojala S, Virkkunen A. Incidence of occult inguinal and spigelian hernias during laparoscopy of other reasons. Surgery. 2006;**140**(1):9-12

[25] Spangen L. Spigelian hernia. World Journal of Surgery. 1989;**13**(5):573-580

[26] Igwe PO, Ibrahim NA. Strangulated sliding spigelian hernia: A case report. International Journal of Surgery Case Reports. 2018;**53**:475-478

[27] Rankin A, Kostusiak M, Sokker A. Spigelian hernia: Case series and review of the literature. Visceral Medicine. 2019;**35**(2):133-136

[28] Mittal T, Kumar V, Khullar R, Sharma A, Soni V, Baijal M, et al. Diagnosis and management of Spigelian hernia: A review of literature and our experience. Journal of Minimal Access Surgery. 2008;**4**(4):95-98

[29] Barnes TG, McWhinnie DL. Laparoscopic Spigelian hernia repair: A systematic review. Surgical Laparoscopy, Endoscopy & Percutaneous Techniques. 2016;**26**(4):265-270

[30] Topal E, Kaya E, Topal NB, Sahin I. Giant spigelian hernia due to abdominal wall injury: A case report. Hernia. 2007;**11**(1):67-69

[31] Larson DW, Farley DR. Spigelian hernias: Repair and outcome for 81 patients. World Journal of Surgery. 2002;**26**(10):1277-1281

[32] Birindelli A, Sartelli M, Di Saverio S, Coccolini F, Ansaloni L, van Ramshorst GH, et al. 2017 update of the WSES guidelines for emergency repair of complicated abdominal wall hernias. World Journal of Emergency Surgery : WJES. 2017;**12**:37

[33] Mizrahi H, Parker MC. Management of asymptomatic inguinal hernia: A systematic review of the evidence. Archives of Surgery. 2012;**147**(3):277-281

[34] Kokotovic D, Sjølander H, Gögenur I, Helgstrand F. Watchful waiting as a treatment strategy for patients with a ventral hernia appears to be safe. Hernia. 2016;**20**(2):281-287

[35] Light D, Chattopadhyay D, Bawa S. Radiological and clinical examination in the diagnosis of Spigelian hernias. Annals of the Royal College of Surgeons of England. 2013;**95**(2):98-100

[36] Applegate WV. Abdominal cutaneous nerve entrapment syndrome (ACNES): A commonly overlooked cause of abdominal pain. The Permanente Journal. Summer 2002;**6**(3):20-27

[37] Weiss Y, Lernau OZ, Nissan S. Spigelian hernia. Annals of Surgery. 1974;**180**(6):836-839

[38] Muysoms FE, Miserez M, Berrevoet F, Campanelli G, Champault GG,

Chelala E, et al. Classification of primary and incisional abdominal wall hernias. Hernia. 2009;**13**(4):407-414

[39] Nagarsheth KH, Nickloes T, Mancini G, Solla JA. Laparoscopic repair of incidentally found Spigelian hernia. JSLS: Journal of the Society of Laparoendoscopic Surgeons. 2011;**15**(1):81-85

[40] Carter JE, Mizes C. Laparoscopic diagnosis and repair of spigelian hernia: Report of a case and technique. American Journal of Obstetrics and Gynecology. 1992;**167**(1):77-78

[41] Henriksen NA, Kaufmann R, Simons MP, Berrevoet F, East B, Fischer J, et al. On behalf of the European hernia society and the Americas hernia society. EHS and AHS guidelines for treatment of primary ventral hernias in rare locations or special circumstances. BJS Open. 2020;**4**(2):342-353

[42] Moreno-Egea A, Carrasco L, Girela E, Martín JG, Aguayo JL, Canteras M. Open vs laparoscopic repair of spigelian hernia: A prospective randomized trial. Archives of Surgery. 2002;**137**(11):1266-1268

[43] Rath A, Bhatia P, Kalhan S, John S, Khetan M, Bindal V, et al. Laparoscopic management of Spigelian hernias. Asian Journal of Endoscopic Surgery. 2013;**6**(3):253-256. DOI: 10.1111/ases.12026

[44] Bittner JG 4th, Edwards MA, Shah MB, MacFadyen BV Jr, Mellinger JD. Mesh-free laparoscopic spigelian hernia repair. The American Surgeon. 2008;**74**(8):713-720

[45] Moreno-Egea A, Campillo-Soto Á, Morales-Cuenca G. Which should be the gold standard laparoscopic technique for handling Spigelian hernias? Surgical Endoscopy. 2015;**29**(4):856-862

[46] Mederos R, Lamas JR, Alvarado J, Matos M, Padron I, Ramos A. Laparoscopic diagnosis and repair of Spigelian hernia: A case report and literature review. International Journal of Surgery Case Reports. 2017;**31**:184-187

[47] Tran H, Tran K, Zajkowska M, Lam V, Hawthorne WJ. Single-incision laparoscopic repair of Spigelian hernia. JSLS. 2015;**19**(1):e2015.001644

[48] Barker R, Gill RS, Brar AS, Birch DW, Karmali S. Emergent laparoscopic repair of a spigelian hernia: Case report and review of the literature. Case Reports in Medicine. 2013;**2013**:197561

[49] Kasirajan K, Lopez J, Lopez R. Laparoscopic technique in the management of Spigelian hernia. Journal of Laparoendoscopic & Advanced Surgical Techniques. Part A. 1997;**7**(6):385-388

[50] Baucom C, Nguyen QD, Hidalgo M, Slakey D. Minimally invasive spigelian hernia repair. JSLS: Journal of the Society of Laparoendoscopic Surgeons. 2009;**13**(2):263-268

[51] Skouras C, Purkayastha S, Jiao L, Tekkis P, Darzi A, Zacharakis E. Laparoscopic management of spigelian hernias. Surgical Laparoscopy, Endoscopy & Percutaneous Techniques. 2011;**21**(2):76-81

[52] Martell EG, Singh NN, Zagorski SM, Sawyer MA. Laparoscopic repair of a spigelian hernia: A case report and literature review. JSLS: Journal of the Society of Laparoendoscopic Surgeons. 2004;**8**(3):269-274

[53] Huber N, Paschke S, Henne-Bruns D, Brockschmidt C. Laparoscopic intraperitoneal mesh fixation with fibrin sealant of a Spigelian hernia. GMS Interdisciplinary Plastic

and Reconstructive Surgery DGPW. 2013;**2**:Doc 08:1-5

[54] Jamshidian M, Stanek S, Sferra J, Jamil T. Robotic repair of symptomatic Spigelian hernias: A series of three cases and surgical technique review. Journal of Robotic Surgery. 2018;**12**(3):557-560

[55] Hanzalova I, Schäfer M, Demartines N, Clerc D. Spigelian hernia: Current approaches to surgical treatment-a review [published online ahead of print, 2021 Oct 19]. Hernia. 2021. DOI: 10.1007/s10029-021-02511-8

[56] Klimopoulos CKAS. Low Spigelian hernias: Experience of 26 consecutive cases in 24 patients. The European Journal of Surgery. 2001;**167**(8):631-633

[57] Basu S, Kumar D, Chaudhury S, Sharma CL. A child with recurrent abdominal pain. ANZ Journal of Surgery. 2007;**77**(12):1133

Chapter 6

Laparoscopic Findings of Rare Pediatric Inguinal Hernias

Michinobu Ohno, Yasushi Fuchimoto, Akihiro Fujino, Toshihiko Watanabe and Yutaka Kanamori

Abstract

Pediatric inguinal hernias are caused to the patency of the processus vaginalis (PPV). The principle for the repair of indirect inguinal hernias in children consists of complete ligation of the PPV. Laparoscopic percutaneous extraperitoneal closure (LPEC) has spread rapidly since it was reported by some groups from around 1998, and the number of institutions adopting this method as a standard procedure for pediatric inguinal hernia is increasing in Japan. Since the closure of PPV by laparoscopic surgery is popular, rare hernias in children can be observed from the abdominal cavity. We present the laparoscopic findings of rare pediatric inguinal hernias and report their experience.

Keywords: indirect inguinal hernia, direct hernia, femoral hernia, child, adult

1. Introduction

Most inguinal hernias in children are classified as indirect inguinal hernias. Laparoscopic percutaneous extraperitoneal closure (LPEC) repair for pediatric indirect inguinal hernia is a standard technique in our facilities [1, 2]. We experienced two rare cases of pediatric inguinal hernias and reported their laparoscopic findings.

2. Case reports

2.1 Case 1

A one-year-old boy was admitted to our hospital for the incarceration of right inguinal hernia several times. He underwent LPEC procedure as a right indirect inguinal hernia. Laparoscopic findings demonstrated that the hernia orifice was present in the medial inguinal fossa (**Figure 1**). We converted the open approach and performed to reinforce the posterior wall of the inguinal canal. After the hernia sac was opened and excised, the transversalis fascia and Cooper's ligament were closed (McVay repair).

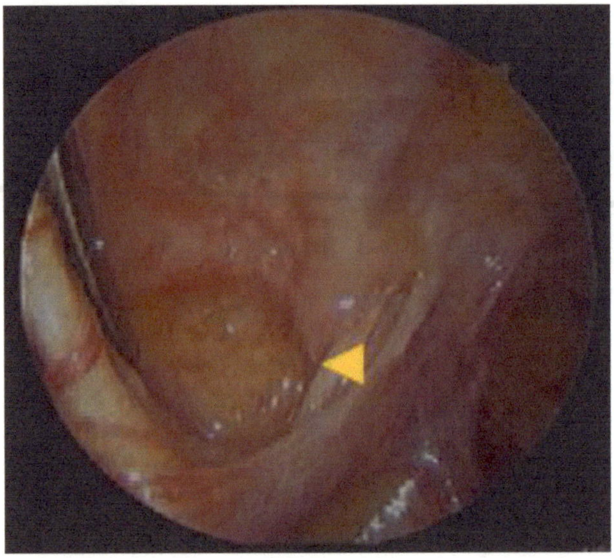

Figure 1.
Laparoscopic finding of right direct inguinal hernia. Hernia orifice presented medially to the external iliac vessels (arrowhead).

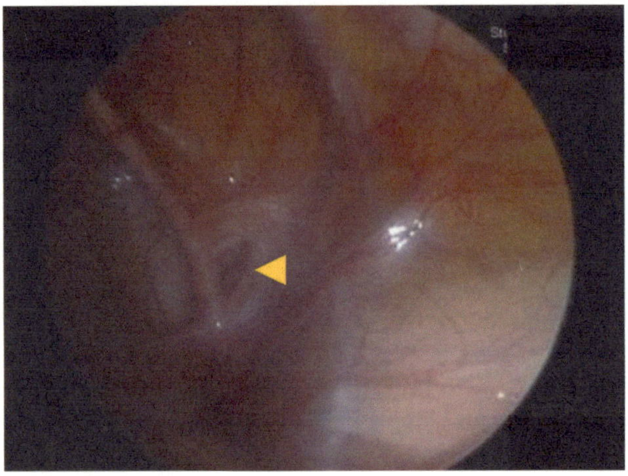

Figure 2.
Laparoscopic finding of femoral hernia at first operation. Hernia orifice presented medially to the epigastric vessels and below the inguinal ligament (arrowhead).

2.2 Case 2

The patient was a seven-year-old girl. She was diagnosed with the right external inguinal hernia and planned for LPEC procedure. Based on laparoscopic findings, we misdiagnosed an internal inguinal hernia (**Figure 2**). Iliopubic tract repair was performed with an open approach. One month after the operation, recurrence of inguinal protrusion was observed, and ultrasonography demonstrated femoral hernia (**Figure 3**). Therefore, the laparoscopic examination was scheduled. Intra-abdominal findings showed that the hernia orifice appeared to be closed, but traction with forceps confirmed the presence of a femoral hernia sac (**Figure 4**).

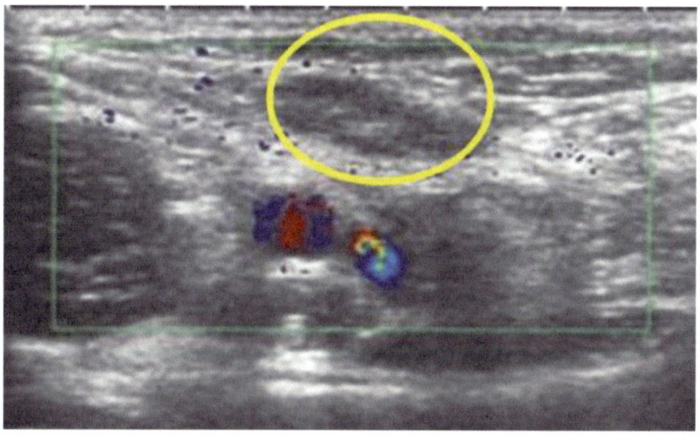

Figure 3.
Ultrasonography of femoral hernia at recurrence. Herniation was recognized caudally to inguinal region and medially to the epigastric vessels (circle).

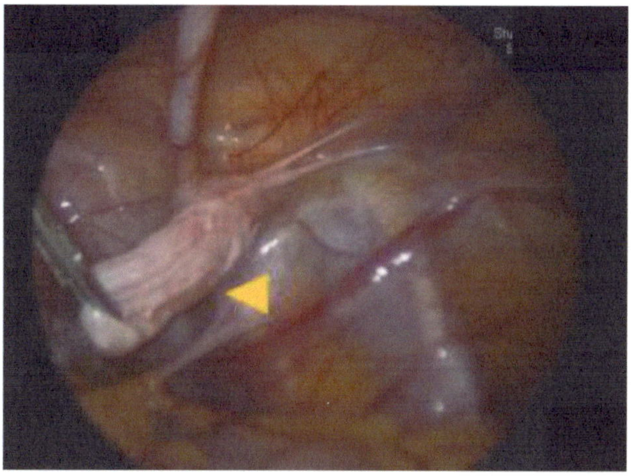

Figure 4.
Laparoscopic finding of femoral hernia at second operation. A hernia sac with fat was identified (arrowhead).

We expected that the second open approach would have strong adhesion, therefore, we chose laparoscopic surgery. The hernia sac with the adipose tissue was resected. The iliopubic tract and Cooper's ligament were exposed and the femoral ring was closed (modified McVay repair).

3. Discussion

Direct inguinal hernia in children is quite rare. The incidence of direct inguinal hernias is as low as 0.2–1.2% of all pediatric inguinal hernias [3, 4]. Direct inguinal hernias seem to occur in males, and the affected side is on the right [4]. Fonkalsrud or other presumed the two or three etiologies of direct inguinal hernia: (1) attenuation of transversalis fascia, (2) increased abdominal pressure, and (3) weakness of the internal inguinal ring due to the previous surgery for indirect inguinal hernia. Wright divides the direct hernia into five based on the findings from the inguinal region [5, 6].

The correct diagnosis rate of indirect inguinal hernia is 38% preoperatively, and diagnosis is often missed even during surgery [5]. Recently, the laparoscopic diagnosis seems to be a feasible choice in this rare condition. In our case, preoperative diagnosis is an indirect inguinal hernia, however laparoscopic findings demonstrated direct hernia during surgery.

The treatment of direct hernia is different in each facility. Some authors recommend Bassini repair [4, 5], and some recommend McVay repair [6]. Laparoscopic closure of indirect hernia is described as an excellent technique for rare hernia. They use the vesical or umbilical ligament to close the direct defect [3, 7, 8]. However, laparoscopic treatment of pediatric inguinal indirect hernia is still controversial, and we performed McVay repair rather than laparoscopic closure to ensure posterior wall reinforcement.

Femoral hernia in children is less than 1% of all groin hernia [9–11]. Previous statements that femoral hernia is equally in males and females [12], and some authors indicated more frequently in boys than girls [13, 14]. A predominance of affected sides reported the right side, however, the cause is not understood [14, 15]. Regarding the etiology of femoral hernia, the most supported hypothesis was described by McVay and Savage [16]. They proposed that a congenital narrow insertion of the posterior inguinal wall onto Cooper's ligament caused an enlargement of the femoral ring.

A femoral hernia is also often misdiagnosed as a direct hernia. The correct diagnosis rate of femoral hernia is 53% preoperatively [17]. Several authors recommended a meticulous physical examination in the inguinal area, and ultrasonography is especially useful to distinguish femoral hernia from indirect inguinal hernia [14, 18]. We misunderstood our case as an indirect inguinal hernia in the first operation. Reconfirming the physical examination, the orifice of hernia was slightly caudal position and ultrasonography demonstrated femoral hernia. Pediatric hernias required a more accurate examination at the first visit.

The advantage of the laparoscopic technique in pediatric hernia includes the accurate diagnosis, minimal pain, and cosmesis. Although laparoscopic repair of femoral hernia was established in adults [19], most pediatric surgeons chose the open approach. In recent years, laparoscopic modified McVay technique reported in children [17, 20]. The laparoscopic approach was performed because of recurrent cases and the possibility of severe adhesion in our case. Laparoscopic closure required more operative time than an open approach. We consider the key to femoral repair is the closure of the hernia orifice without tension, following the resection of lipoma with the hernia sac.

4. Conclusions

Numerous pediatric surgeons have never seen rare hernias, however, in the laparoscopic era, intraabdominal findings revealed more higher rate of rare hernias. Rare pediatric inguinal hernias are challenging to diagnose and treat. In our both cases, the laparoscope approach was useful for diagnosis, however, simple or modified laparoscopic closure is still controversial.

Acknowledgements

I am grateful to Yuko Nakamura and Yuka Nomura for cooperating and supporting me as a medical team.

Conflict of interest

The authors declare no conflict of interest.

Notes/thanks/other declarations

Thanks to my colleagues.

Acronyms and abbreviations

PPV	patency of the processus vaginalis
LPEC	laparoscopic percutaneous extraperitoneal closure

Author details

Michinobu Ohno[1*], Yasushi Fuchimoto[2], Akihiro Fujino[3], Toshihiko Watanabe[4] and Yutaka Kanamori[3]

1 Department of Pediatric Surgery, Saitama City Hospital, Saitama, Japan

2 Department of Pediatric Surgery, International University of Health and Welfare, Narita, Japan

3 Division of Surgery, National Center for Child Health and Development, Tokyo, Japan

4 Department of Pediatric Surgery, Tokai University, Isehara, Japan

*Address all correspondence to: mohnomohno2000@hotmail.co.jp

IntechOpen

© 2022 The Author(s). Licensee IntechOpen. This chapter is distributed under the terms of the Creative Commons Attribution License (http://creativecommons.org/licenses/by/3.0), which permits unrestricted use, distribution, and reproduction in any medium, provided the original work is properly cited. (cc) BY

References

[1] Endo M, Ukiyama E. Laparoscopic closure of patent processus vaginalis in girls with inguinal hernia using a specially devised suture needle. Pediatric Endosurgery & Innovative Techniques. 2001;**5**:187-191

[2] Takehara H, Yakabe H, Kameoka K. Laparoscopic percutaneous extracorponeal closure for inguinal hernia in children: Clinical outcome of 972 repairs done in 3 pediatric surgical institutions. Journal of Pediatric Surgery. 2006;**41**:1999-2003

[3] Schier F. Direct inguinal hernias in children: Laparoscopic aspects. Pediatric Surgery International. 2000;**16**(8):562-564

[4] Wright JE. Direct inguinal hernia in infancy and childhood. Pediatric Surgery International. 1994;**9**:161-163

[5] Fonkalsrud EW, Delorimier AA, Clatworthy HW Jr. Femoral and direct inguinal hernias in infants and children. JAMA. 1965;**192**:597-599

[6] Viidik T, Marshall DG. Direct inguinal hernias in infancy and early childhood. Journal of Pediatric Surgery. 1980;**15**(5):646-647

[7] Esposito C, Montinaro L, Alicchio F, Scermino S, Basile A, Armenise T, et al. Technical standardization of laparoscopic herniorraphy in pediatric patients. World Journal of Surgery. 2009;**33**(9):1846-1850

[8] Lima M, Ruggeri G, Domini M, Lauro V, Libri M, Bertozzi M. Laparoscopic treatment of bilateral direct inguinal hernia by using the vesical ligament as an autologous patch. Pediatric Endosurgery & Innovative Techniques. 2002;**4**:277-280

[9] Fosburg RG, Marlin HP. Femoral hernia in children. American Journal of Surgery. 1965;**109**:470-475

[10] Marshall DG. Femoral hernia in children. Journal of Pediatric Surgery. 1983;**18**:160-162

[11] Schier R, Klizaite J. Rare inguinal heria forms in children. Pediatric Surgery International. 2004;**20**:748-752

[12] Donnellan WL. Inguinal and femoral hernias. In: Donnellan WL, Burrington JD, Kimura K, editors. Abdominal Surgery of Infancy and Childhood. Luxemburg: Harwood; 1996. pp. 52/16-52/18

[13] Temiz A, Akcora B, Temiz M, et al. A rare and frequently unrecognised pathology in children: Femoral hernia. Hernia. 2008;**12**:553-556

[14] Aneiros Castro B, Cano Novillo I, García Vázquez A, López Díaz M, Benavent Gordo MI, Gómez Fraile A. Pediatric femoral hernia in the laparoscopic era. Asian Journal of Endoscopic Surgery. 2018;**11**(3):233-237

[15] Wright MF, Scollay JM, McCabe AJ, et al. Paediatric femoral hernia: The diagnostic challenge. International Journal of Surgery. 2011;**9**:472-474

[16] McVay CB, Savage LE. Etiology of femoral hernia. Annals of Surgery. 1961;**154**:25-32

[17] De Caluwe D, Chertin B, Puri P. Childhood femoral hernia: A commonly misdiagnosed condition. Pediatric Surgery International. 2003;**19**:608-609

[18] Erez I, Rathause V, Vacian I, et al. Preoperative ultrasound and

intraoperative findings of inguinal hernias in children: A prospective study of 642 children. Journal of Pediatric Surgery. 2002;**37**:865-868

[19] Peitsch WK. A modified laparoscopic hernioplasty (TAPP) is the standard procedure for inguinal and femoral hernias: A retrospective 17-year analysis with 1123 hernia repairs. Surgical Endoscopy. 2014;**28**:671-682

[20] Tainaka T, Uchida H, Ono Y, Tanano A, Shirota C, Yokota K, et al. A new modification of laparoscopic percutaneous extraperitoneal closure procedure for repairing pediatric femoral hernias involving a special needle and a wire loop. Nagoya Journal of Medical Science. 2015;77(3):531-535

Chapter 7

Transabdominal Preperitoneal (TAPP) Inguinal Hernia Repair

Giovambattista Caruso, Giuseppe Evola, Salvatore Antonio Maria Benfatto and Mariapia Gangemi

Abstract

The inguinal hernia repair is one of the most frequent surgical procedures: in the world, even year, at least 20.000.000 inguinal hernia repair procedures are performed. Although the laparoscopic approach is widely recognized as a valid treatment for many diseases and some laparoscopic surgical procedures have become gold standard techniques (e. g. cholecystectomy, appendectomy, gastro-esophageal junction surgery), the minimally invasive approach for groin hernia treatment is still very controversial today, but in the last few years, it tends to become the standard practice for 1 day surgery. We present here the technique of laparoscopic Transabdominal Preperitoneal approach (TAPP). The surgical technique is described step-by-step, including surgical details and the new concept of "inverted Y" to achieve the "critical view of safety" for laparoscopic inguinal hernia repair.

Keywords: TAPP, inguinal hernia, minimally invasive surgery, transabdominal preperitoneal approach, laparoscopy

1. Introduction

Inguinal hernia repair is one of the most frequent surgical procedures performed around the world; around 20 million hernioplasties are done every year. However, although laparoscopic inguinal hernia repair was initiated more than 28 years ago, most hernioplasties are still performed with an open approach [1]. Although the laparoscopic approach is widely recognized as a valid treatment for many diseases and some laparoscopic surgical procedures have become gold standard techniques (e. g. cholecystectomy, appendectomy, gastro-esophageal junction surgery), the minimally invasive approach for groin hernia treatment is still very controversial today. The main pretexts are the higher costs, the use of general anesthesia and the possible higher rate of major complications associated with laparoscopic procedures. Another reticence related to laparoscopic approach is the greater surgical complexity linked to need to recognize a "new" anatomy of the posterior inguinal wall, which is still unusual for general surgeons. Much more the choice of laparoscopic approach (TransAbdominal PrePeritoneal (TAPP) versus Totally Extraperitoneal (TEP)) is also controversial [2]. We present herein the TAPP procedure focusing on tips and tricks for better outcomes [3].

2. Anatomy

The abdominal wall is an uneven area with natural openings and areas of weakness that can be the site of hernias formed by the externalization of a peritoneal sac that can contain viscera. The inguinal area has a complex anatomical entity, due to its configuration, it constitutes the passage of intra-abdominal elements toward the outside. This is the starting point for all hernias.

The inguinal area is the main weak point of the anterior abdominal wall and corresponds to the pectineus orifice, embryologically weakened by the passage of the spermatic cord in men (inguinal canal) and of the femoral vessels (femoral canal).

Perfect knowledge of the anatomy of the groin region is the key to treating hernias. Several works have been dedicated to this region with evidence of a natural parietal weakness. According to recent studies on the anatomy of the groin area, Fruchaud has confirmed that all inguinal hernias pass through a single parietal orifice called the myopectineal orifice delimited medially by rectus abdominis muscle, inferiorly by pectineum ligament, laterally by Psoas muscle and superiorly by Transversus Abdominis and Internal oblique muscle (Transverse arch). The inguinal ligament passes over this structure dividing it into two portions, the inguinal region above (crossed by the spermatic cord) and the crural region below (crossed by femoral vessels). It is internally covered by the transverse fascia only. Observed from inside the abdomen with the peritoneum intact, the lower part of the anterior abdominal wall is usually divided into three fossae, separated by the same number of folds or ligaments formed by different protruding structures. On the median line we identify the Urachus, also called median umbilical ligament. Lateral to the Urachus we find the lateral umbilical ligament, usually the most evident of the three folds. The ligament is a remnant of the umbilical artery, now obliterated, which leads from the iliac artery toward the navel. Finally, the outermost fold, corresponding to the inferior epigastric vessels, is the least protruding. The most common classification of the inguinal hernias still uses these three folds as lanmarks. Indirect inguinal hernias are those that originate laterally to the epigastric vessels, direct inguinal hernias are those medial to them, and the supravesical hernias are those originate between the median and umbilical ligaments. Femoral hernias are located below this plane, below the iliopubic tract and through a space around the femoral sheath. On very rare occasions, obturator hernias are found, linked to a defect of the obturate membrane of the iliac bone. Through the intact parietal peritoneum, it is possible to recognize the round ligament in women and the vas deferens in men. Both proceed obliquely from the deep part of the pelvis upwards and from inside to the outside, to emerge from the abdomen through the internal inguinal orifice crossing the epigastric vessels. The transabdominal preperitoneal laparoscopic hernioplasty requires the preparation of a very large peritoneal flap. To do this, it is very important to know how to recognize and identify the extraperitoneal spaces of the pelvis. Medially, between the parietal peritoneum and the transversalis fascia, is the Retzius space, consisting of variable amount of adipose tissue. It is usually an avascular space except in the lower part where there are venous anastomoses between the epigastric, obturate and iliopubic vessels. Although the inguinal ligament is not visible, however, Cooper's ligament is visible and palpable with laparoscopic instruments even in obese subjects. This important reference point is located 1 cm medial and inferior to the origin of the epigastric vessels [4].

In males, the spermatic vessels join an obtuse angle with the deferent conduct, and also exit through the internal inguinal orifice, to form outside it, with the the fasciae and muscular fibers enveloping it, the spermatic cord.

The *Inverted Y* created with inferior epigastric vessels (superiorly), vas deferens (medially) and spermatic vessels (laterally) allows to better understand and recognize the anatomical structures.

Recognition of these elements, in fact, is the basis for understanding the technical steps for repairs all types of inguinal hernias by laparoscopy.

The inferior epigastric vessels separate the medial and lateral inguinal regions, permitting the classification of direct inguinal hernias (collapse of the transversalis fascia, medially to the epigastric vessels), and indirect (enlargement of deep inguinal ring, laterally to the epigastric vessels).

Another important anatomical landmark is the iliopubic tract, which represents the intra-abdominal view of the inguinal ligament. It extends from the anterosuperior iliac crest to the pectineum (Cooper's) ligament and separates the superior and inferior inguinal spaces. The upper portion is the point of onset of inguinal hernias (direct, indirect, mixed, supravesical). Femoral or crural hernias, as well as the obturators, originate in the lower portion of the inguinal space, below the iliopubic tract.

Identification of inverted Y elements and iliopubic tract, that passes horizontally through the deep inguinal ring at the center of the inverted Y, permit visualization of five areas (*the Five Triangles*) (**Figure 1**).

Disaster or *Doom triangle,* formed by vas deferens, medially, and spermatic vessels, laterally, it corresponds to the location of the external iliac vessels.

Pain triangle (or of the nerves), delimited, medially, by spermatic vessels and, laterally and superiorly, by iliopubic tract; it represents the passage of lateral cutaneous nerve of the thigh, femoral branch of the genitofemoral nerve and femoral nerve.

Triangle of Indirect hernias: correspond to the deep inguinal ring, the source of indirect hernias. It is formed by inferior epigastric vessels, medially, and by iliopubic tract inferiorly and laterally.

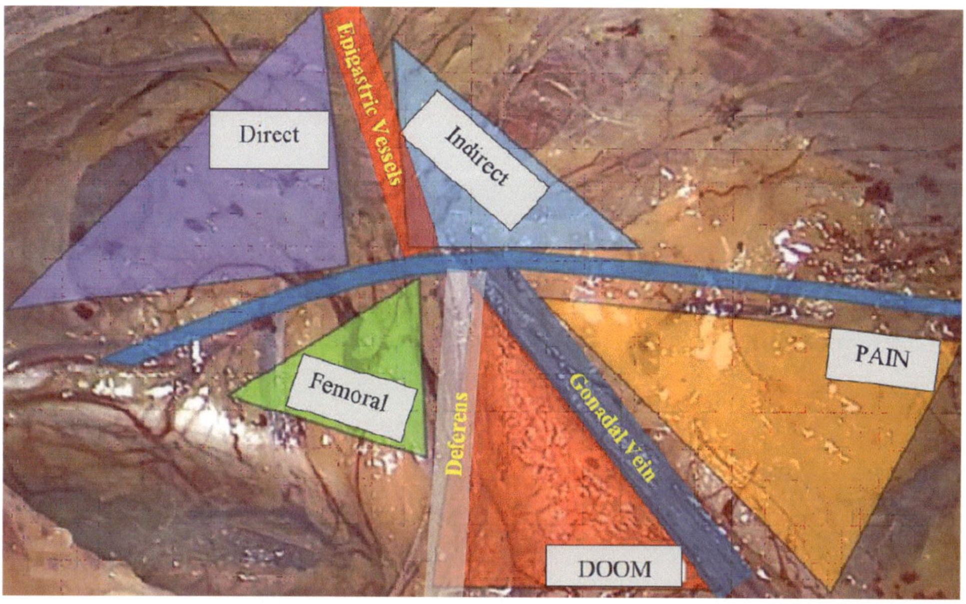

Figure 1.
The Inverted Y *and the* Five Triangles.

Hesselbach's triangle or direct hernias: delimited medially by lateral border of the rectus abdominis muscle, laterally by the inferior epigastric vessels, inferiorly by the iliopubic tract. It is the site of occurrence of direct hernias.

Triangle of Femoral hernias: is not a true triangle but identifies the area corresponding to the ostium of the femoral vein, delimited, at the top, by iliopubic tract, laterally by the external iliac vein, at the bottom by pectineum ligament and medially by the lacunar ligament.

This didactic way of posterior visualization of the miopectineal orifice, defining the inverted Y and the five triangles, facilitates the anatomical understanding of inguinocrural region and of all hernia defects that may occur [5].

3. Indications and contraindications

With very few exceptions the TAPP approach can be performed in theory for any hernia, even in strangulated or incarcerated cases; however, the indication depends on the surgeon's clinical judgment and skills. The best indications according to Nyhus classification are:

- Type 3 and 4 hernias
- Bilateral hernias
- Hernias in obese patients
- Hernias in subjects with intense physical activity (sport, strenuous working)
- Recurrence of hernia after open repairs.

They are very few contraindications for these procedures, such as:

- Intolerance to capnoperitoneum (severe cardiopathies or severe pneumopathies)
- Extensive intra-abdominal adhesion
- Large scrotal hernia
- After radical prostatectomy
- Strangulated or perforated hernia with intercurrent sepsis
- Severe ascites
- Recurrence of hernia after laparoscopic repair
- Pediatric patients
- Pregnancy after the second trimester
- Severe clotting disorders

4. Preoperative preparation

The patient has to be carefully prepared for the operation. The evaluation of comorbidities as well as an adequate skin preparation is mandatory. The patient has to be informed about the details of the surgical procedure and the possible negative outcomes, as the latest guidelines recommended [6].

4.1 Evaluation of the operative risk

Using ASA (American Society of Anesthetist) Score. From the point of view of comorbidities, there are no "absolute" contraindications for TAPP. The anticoagulant oral therapy is replaced by low molecular weight heparins (LMWH) and the procedure is usually performed at least 12 hours after the last LMWH dose. The new anticoagulant oral drugs (e. g. Dabigatran etexilate - Pradaxa®; Apixaban - Eliquis®; Rivaroxaban - Xarelto®) is stopped and replaced by LMWH at least 5 days before the procedure. Clopidogrel or ticlopidine are stopped and replaced by aspirin 5 to 7 days before the procedure and higher doses of aspirin are reduced to 75 mg/day 3 to 7 days before the procedure [7].

4.2 Skin preparation

a preoperative antiseptic shower is performed on the eve of the intervention. The hair is removed, half an hour before the surgery, from middle thorax until the upper third of the things using an electric barber clipper. Alcohol based solutions (Iodine or Chlorexidine gluconate in case of iodine allergy) are used for skin preparation after anesthetic induction [8].

4.3 Urinary Catheter

Always empty the bladder to facilitate the dissection in the Retzius space and to avoid bladder injuries. In selected cases (e. g. bilateral hernia, recurrent hernia), a urinary catheter can be left throughout the surgery [6].

4.4 Patient and surgical team position

The patient is placed in the supine position, with both arms along the body and fixed to the operating table. At the start of the surgery a Trendelemburg position (15–20°) is given eith lateral inclination opposite to the hernial defect. The surgical team is organized with the surgery on the contralateral side to the hernia to be repaired and the camera operator is positioned on the same side, or in the side as the hernia. The scrub nurse stands in front of the surgeon near the patient's feet. In case of bilateral inguinal hernioplasty, the surgical team switch positions when they have finished the first hernia (**Figure 2**). In case of bilateral hernioplasty it is preferable to use a column with two monitors; this is to avoid changing of the laparoscopic column between one side and the other [9].

4.5 Anesthesia

Although we have reported successful cases of laparoscopic inguinal hernioplasty under anesthesia with peridural blockade and sedation, as a general rule we prefer

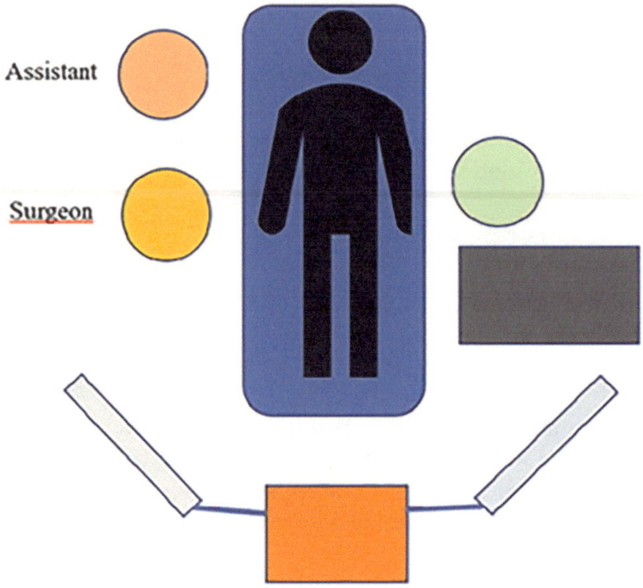

Figure 2.
Surgical team position.

general anesthesia for the patient, as muscle relaxation improves surgical maneuvers and, again, orotracheal intubation protects the airways from vomiting or regurgitation favored by increased intra-abdominal pressure. The preoperative antibiotic prophylaxis (single dose of Cefazoline 2 g during anesthetic induction) is reserved in presence of high-risk factors for wound infection based on patient (recurrence, advanced age, immune deficiency) or surgical (forecast of long surgical intervention, use of drains) factors [10].

4.6 Laparoscopic instruments

Three trocars are necessary, one of 10 mm (optical) and two of 5 mm (for the instruments), as well as common laparoscopic instruments (monopolar scissor, monopolar hook, two atraumatic fenestrated graspers, needle holder, 5 mm Endo peanut, 5 mm disposable absorbable screw type stapler device) and "open surgery" instruments (two Kelly, two Halsted, Farabeuf retractors, scissors and Hegar needle holder). A bipolar grasper and a suction-irrigation device could be also necessary. Usually we use a 30° laparoscope, but a 0° is also feasible.

5. Surgical procedure

5.1 Pneumoperitoneum and trocar placement

Although many surgeons create pneumoperitoneum with Verres needle, we prefer an open technique, using a 10 mm Hasson trocar, through an upper horizontal paraumbilical incision. This incision gives us excellent esthetic results. Under direct vision, two additional 5 mm operating trocars are placed in each flank, in a horizontal plane with the umbilicus. It must be remembered that a small number of patients present with a contralateral hernia although not diagnosed preoperatively. This trocars position is convenient for both unilateral and bilateral hernias (**Figure 3**).

5.2 Abdominal Exploration

The aim of the laparoscopic exploration is to identify the superficial anatomical landmarks (Urachus, umbilical folds, epigastric vessels, spermatic vessels, vas deferens or uterine round ligament) and the site and type of hernia. The two "dangerous triangles", vascular and pain triangles, must be correctly identified [2]. To perform the exploration and to ensure a good exposure of the inguinal region the position of the operating table is kept in 15° Trendelemburg with 15° lateral rotation to the side opposite the hernia (**Figure 4**).

5.3 Peritoneal incision

The TAPP procedure starts with peritoneal cut 2 cm above and 1 cm medial from the anterior superior iliac spine and continue horizontally, in medial direction to the lateral umbilical ligament (umbilical artery), then the incision continues vertically along the umbilical ligament, using the monopolar hook or scissors (**Figure 5**). This creates an "L" shape incision. After the first peritoneal cut, the CO2 peumoperitoneum will enter into the preperitoneal space, facilitating the dissection [11].

5.4 Dissection of lower Peritoneal Flap

The aim of this step is to create a preperitoneal pocket to ensure the best positioning of the mesh. This step consists of three phases: 1) Medial dissection over the Retzius space, 2) Lateral dissection on the space of Bogros, 3) Central dissection over the site of the hernia and its hernial sac. We usually start with the medial dissection (Retzius space), dividing the conjunctive fibers in contact with the rectus abdominal

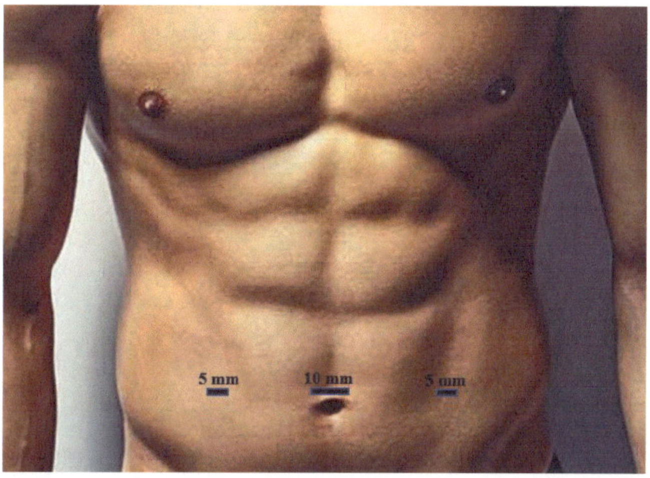

Figure 3.
Trocar's position.

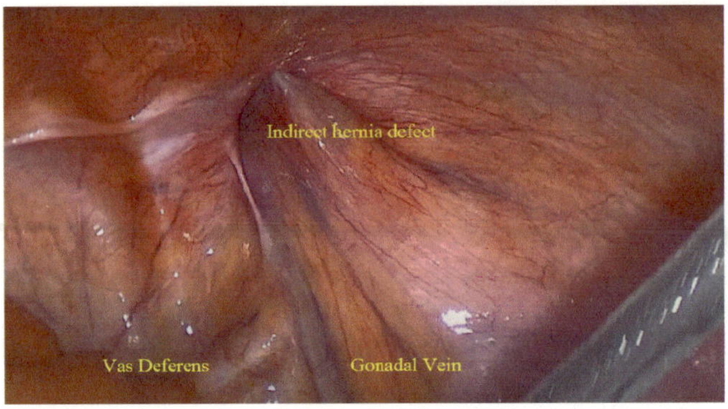

Figure 4.
The intra-abdominal view.

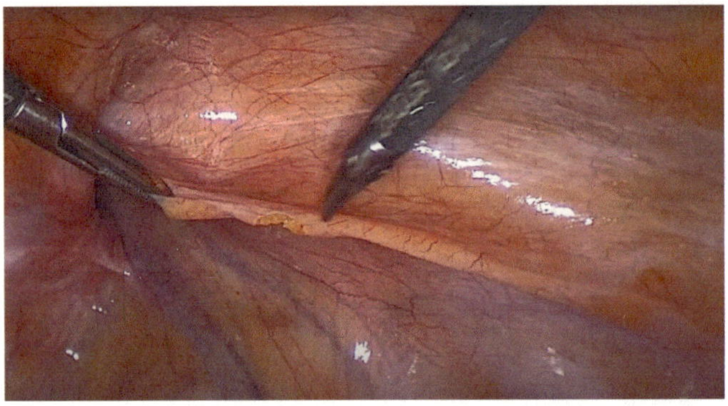

Figure 5.
Peritoneum incision.

muscle to avoid bladder injuries; this way the bladder is detached from the abdominal rectus muscles. The dissection is conducted to the pubis to expose Cooper's ligament (**Figures 6**, 7), which we almost invariably find on dissecting 1 cm medial and 1 cm inferior to the origin of the deep epigastric vessels. Usually, in contact with the pubic bone there are several fine vessels originated from the corona mortis. We prefer to

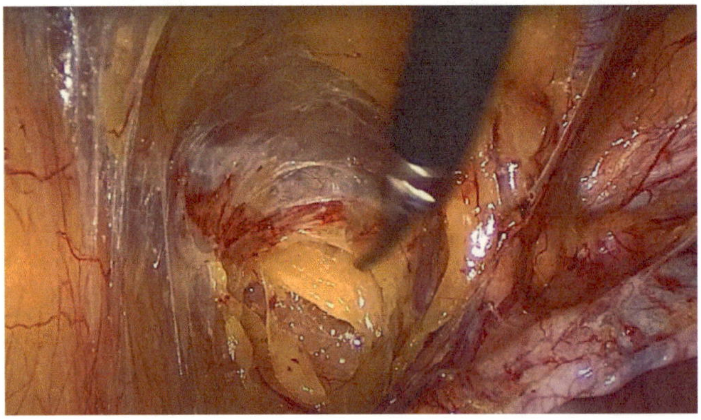

Figure 6.
Medial dissection.

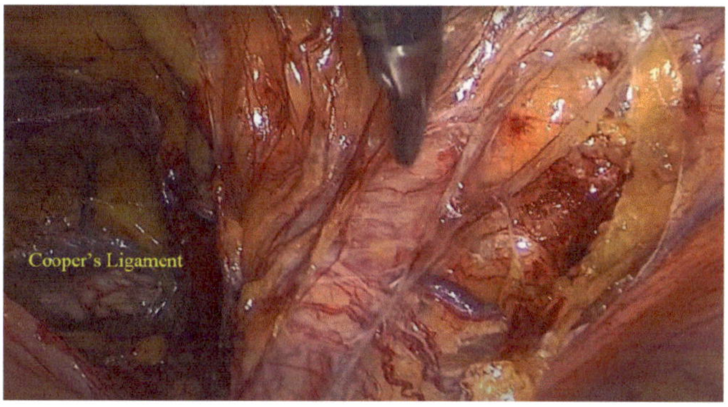

Figure 7.
Medial dissection.

coagulate them to avoid further bleeding during the dissection or mesh stapling. The dissection is then conducted laterally on the space of Bogros, tractioning the peritoneum in the medial direction, from the epigastric vessels until the spermatic vessels (**Figure 8**). The sac dissection is performed using traction contra-traction maneuvers and fine coagulation. To avoid the injuries of the ductus deferens and spermatic vessels the sac dissection always starts anteriorly (**Figures 9, 10**). To facilitate dissection of the peritoneal flap, endo peanuts can be helped. When the hernia sac is very large, we prefer to cut and leave it in situ. This avoids the risk of involuntary injury to the elements of the spermatic cord, reducing the risk of ischemic orchitis, inguino-scrotal hematoma and/or testicular atrophy. However, the incidence of inguino-scrotal seroma or "pseudo-hydrocele" is higher when this maneuver is adopted. We always check for hernia lipoma as recommended in the literature [6]. It is necessary to extend the dissection caudally to the obturator fossa to identify eventual occult obturator hernia especially in women. The preperitoneal dissection ends when the anatomic landmarks previous described are well exposed and the two dangerous triangles (vascular and of the pain) can be identified (**Figure 11**). For large parietal defects, the transversalis fascia has to be inverted and stapled to the Cooper ligament. This simple maneuver seems to decrease the postoperative seroma rate [12].

5.5 Mesh placement

One of the most issues in the laparoscopic approach to inguinal hernioplasty is the need to use a prosthetic mesh to fully cover the hernial defect and all possible herniation sites in the area. The mesh should reach at least the pubic symphysis medially and the iliopsoas muscle laterally. Inferiorly it should reach 1–2 cm below the pubis and superiorly cover the anterior abdominal wall, exceeding the hernial defect by 3–4 cm. We usually use a large "anatomical pre-shaped" (12 x 15 cm) polypropylene mesh which is inserted from the optical trocar. The prosthesis is rolled up on its long side and grasping it with the grasper at the medial end is easily introduced through the Hasson into the abdomen. The medial end of the prosthesis is brought over the Cooper. The prosthesis is then unrolled and the medial head is anchored to the Cooper with the absorbable tacking staples, taking care not to injure the "corona mortis vessels" (**Figure 12**). This first tack facilitates further unrolling of the prosthesis and its placement in the preperitoneal pocket and fixation, with the absorbable tacking staples, on the upper and medial edge, as well as at the level of the iliac

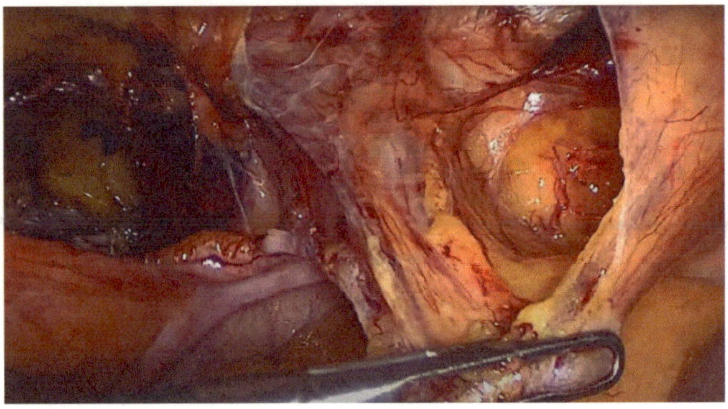

Figure 8.
Lateral dissection.

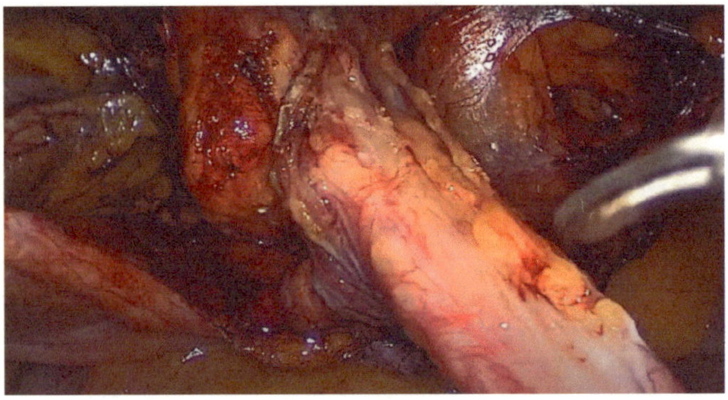

Figure 9.
Sac dissection.

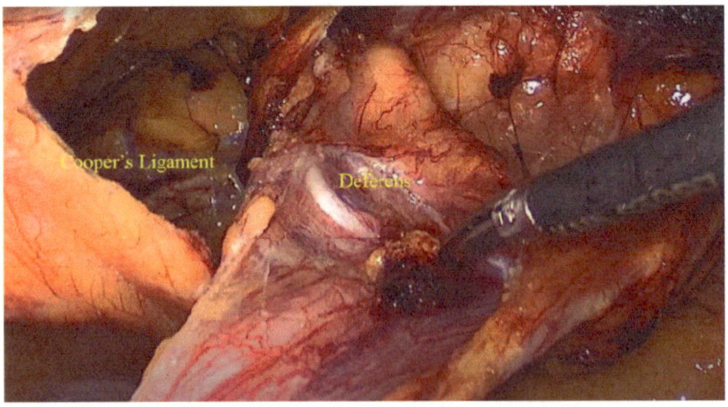

Figure 10.
Sac dissection.

spine (**Figures 13, 14**). Some alternatives to staple fixation are noted in the literature: the use of fibrin glue [13], the self-gripping mesh [14], trans parietal sutures [15], or, even, the recent no fixation technique [16]. For bilateral hernia we use two separate meshes covering the bilateral defects overlapping and stapled together on the median line; this technique is easier than the deployment of one single large mesh.

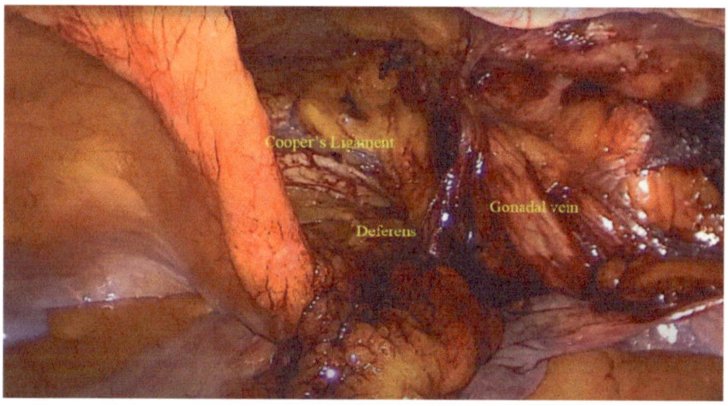

Figure 11.
Intraoperative inverted Y.

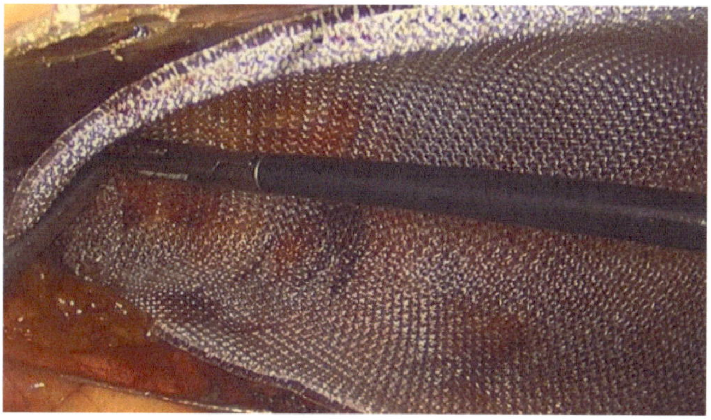

Figure 12.
Mesh fixation to Cooper's ligament.

5.6 Drainage

Some authors emphasize the role of suction-draining in decreasing postoperative seroma and hematoma rates, as the release of carbon dioxide pressure is followed by bleeding from capillaries. We use 24 hours suction-drainage for selected cases: difficult dissection, anticoagulant or antiplatelet therapy, intraoperative hemorrage, partial hernial sac resection [17].

5.7 Peritoneal closure

Our routine is to close the peritoneal flap with the aid of helicoidal absorbable tacks. This maneuver is fast and cost-effective. Alternatively, we also close the flap with continuous suture (2–0 monofilament or 3–0 barbed suture) (**Figure 15**). Before start the peritoneal closure, we lower capnoperitoneum pressure to 8 mmHg to facilitate the approximation of the edges of the peritoneum under less tension [6, 11, 16].

5.8 Abdominal closure

After the careful examination of the peritoneal closure, the trocars are removed under laparoscopic control. The aponevrosis is closed at umbilical site with a purse

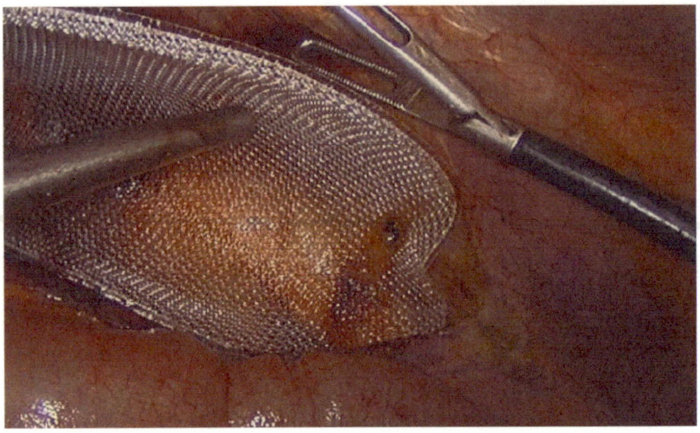

Figure 13.
Lateral fixation of the mesh.

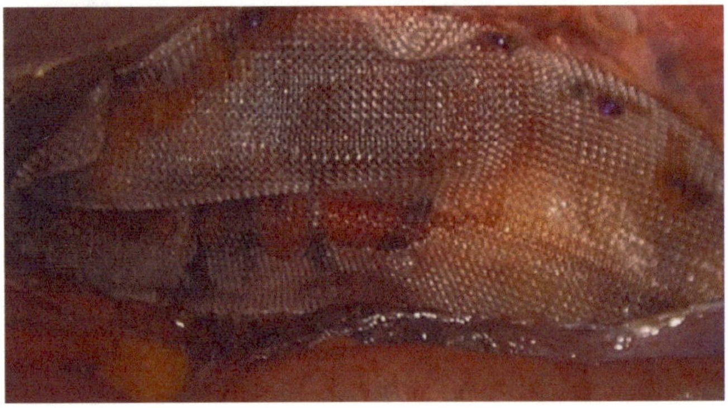

Figure 14.
Implanted mesh.

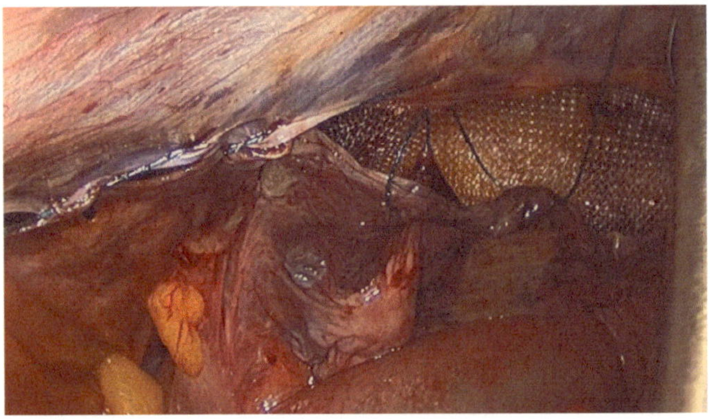

Figure 15.
Peritoneum closure.

string suture with absorbable suture. The operative wounds are infiltrated with long-acting anesthetics (Levobupivacaine) for a better control of postoperative pain. Alternatively, the laparoscopic TAP Block can be used. The skin is closed using inverted fast absorbable sutures or staples.

5.9 Intraoperative complications

Intraoperative bleeding is one of the potential complications of TAPP. The injuries of the deep epigastric vessels, the testicular artery, the gonadal veins or the corona mortis can cause abundant bleeding which, if not controllable by laparoscopy, require immediate conversion to open. Obviously, the lesion of the iliac vessels requires an immediate conversion to laparotomy for vascular control and the relative repair of the damage.

6. Postoperative management

The immediate postoperative analgesic therapy consists in Paracetamol 1000 mg × 3/day and Ketoralac 30 mg IV × 2/day. The urinary catheter, if placed, is removed 6 hours after surgery. As soon as the general conditions allow it, the patient is mobilized and invited to walk. The in-hospital stay is 24 hours (Day Surgery). A liquid diet is indicated 4 hours after surgery. We perform a routine thromboembolic disease prophylaxis with low molecular weight heparins (LMWH) therapy for 7 days, for all the patients. We recommend using an ice pack over the repaired groin for the first 48 hours after surgery and maintaining the use of a hernia support tensor for 4–6 weeks. At home, patients continue taking oral analgesic as necessary (Paracetamol, Ketoprofen).

Light physical activity is recommended (walking, slowly climbing one or two flights of stairs) from the first day after surgery, regular physical activity (walks and resumption of work that does not require strenuous physical exertion) is allowed from day 7 or 10, and intense physical activity only from the fourth week after surgery.

In the consulting room, we examine the patients around 7 days after surgery, then 1 month after surgery, and then every 6 months for long-term follow-up.

7. Postoperative complications

These include seromas, hematomas, postoperative chronic pain, infection of wounds, rejection or infection of the mesh, postoperative adherential syndrome, recurrences, testicular atrophy and infertility.

Seroma is the only complication more frequent in laparoscopic technique than in open repairs. While the rate of this complication is about 5.7% in the literature, we reported a 5% rate. Only in voluminous seroma is recommended the aspiration or drainage.

Hematoma is less frequent in laparoscopic hernia repair than in open repairs, with a rate of about 8% and rarely requires drainage or transfusions. In hour experience, hematoma was reported in only 0,8% cases.

Chronic pain, defined as persistence of pain 3 months after the operation, is less frequent after TAPP and is related to tack stapled nerve damage. To date no cases of chronic pain in our experience.

The recurrence rate is described between 0.4 and 4.8% and correlates with the degree of experience of the surgeon. A significant and repeated increase in intra-abdominal pressure appears to be the predisposing factor for relapses. In case of recurrence, guidelines recommend open repair, however, many experienced surgeons are able to treat relapses laparoscopically without any problems.

8. Conclusion

TAPP is associated with a better immediate postoperative comfort, less chronic pain and numbness, less mesh infection, as well as a faster return to usual activities. Another advantage of the laparoscopic technique is the possibility of diagnose and to treat during the same operation the occult hernias. The disadvantages of laparoscopic procedures are longer learning curve with higher risk of complications during the first 30–50 procedures and higher direct costs (general anesthesia, laparoscopic equipment, staples); this costs can be recuperated decreasing the indirect costs: shorter hospital stay and faster return to work.

Conflict of interest

The authors declare no conflict of interest.

Author details

Giovambattista Caruso[1]*, Giuseppe Evola[2], Salvatore Antonio Maria Benfatto[1] and Mariapia Gangemi[3]

1 SS. Salvatore Hospital Paternò (ASP Catania), Italy

2 ARNAS Garibaldi Catania, Italy

3 Policlinico Universitario Catania, Italy

*Address all correspondence to: carusogb@inwind.it

IntechOpen

© 2022 The Author(s). Licensee IntechOpen. This chapter is distributed under the terms of the Creative Commons Attribution License (http://creativecommons.org/licenses/by/3.0), which permits unrestricted use, distribution, and reproduction in any medium, provided the original work is properly cited.

References

[1] Rivas JF et al. Transabdominal preperitoneal (TAPP) inguinal hernia repair: How we do it. Laparoscopic and Endoscopic Surgery. 2020;**6**:1-6

[2] Moldovanu R et al. Laparoscopic transabdominal pre-peritoneal (TAPP) for bilateral inguinal hernia. Jurnalul de Chirurgie, Iasi. 2010;**6**(3):373-382

[3] Moldovanu R, Pavy G. Laparoscopic transabdominal pre-preperitoneal (TAPP) procedure – step-by-step tips and tricks. Chirurgia. 2014;**109**:407-415

[4] Arregui ME. Surgical anatomy of the preperitoneal fasciae, and posterior trasversalis fasciae in the inguinal region. Hernia. 1997;**1**:101-110

[5] Furtado M et al. Systemization of laparoscopic inguinal hernia repair (TAPP) based on a new anatomical concept: inverted Y and five triangles. ABCD Arq Bras Cir Dig. 2019;**32**(1):e1426

[6] Bittner R, Arregui ME, Bisgaard D, Dudai M, Ferzli GS, Fitzgibbons RJ, et al. Guidelines for laparoscopic (TAPP) and endoscopic (TEP) treatment of inguinal hernia. Surgical Endoscopy. 2011;**25**(9):2773-2843

[7] Joubert F, Gillois P, Bouaziz H, Marret E, Iohom G, Albaladejo P. Bleeding complications following peripheral regional anaesthesia in patients treated with anticoagulants or antiplatelet agents: A systematic review. Anaesthesia Critical Care & Pain Medicine. 2019;**38**(5):507-516

[8] Tanner J, Moncaster K, Woodings D. Preoperative hair removal: A systematic review. Journal of Perioperative Practice. 2007;**17**(3):118-121 124-132

[9] Petro CC, Prabhu AS. Preoperativ planning and patient optimization. The Surgical Clinics of North America. 2018;**98**:483-497

[10] Martin C et al. Antibioprophylaxis in surgery and interventional medicine (adult patients). Update 2017. Anaesthesia Critical Care & Pain Medicine. 2019;**38**(5):549-562

[11] Leroy J. Transabdominal preperitoneal approach (TAPP). 2001; 1(3). Available from: https://websurg.com/en/doi/vd01en2173/

[12] Reddy VM, Sutton CD, Bloxham L, Garcea G, Ubhi SS, Robertson GS. Laparoscopic repair of direct inguinal hernia: a new technique that reduces the development of postoperative seroma. Hernia. 2007;**11**(5):393-396 Epub 2007 Jun 1

[13] Lau H. Fibrin sealant versus mechanical stapling for mesh fixation during endoscopic extraperitoneal inguinal hernioplasty: A randomized prospective trial. Annals of Surgery. 2005;**242**(5):670-675

[14] Fumagalli R et al. Self-gripping mesh versus staple fixation in laparoscopic inguinal hernia repair: A prospective comparison. Surgical Endoscopy. 2013;**27**(5):1798-1802

[15] Abdelhamid MS. Transabdominal pre-peritoneal inguinal hernia repair with external fixation. Hernia. 2011;**15**(2):185-188 Epub 2011 Feb 11

[16] Memon MA et al. Laparoscopic inguinal hernia repair: Transabdominal Preperitoneale (TAPP) and Totally Extraperitoneal (TEP). In: Scott-Conner

(CEH), editor. The SAGES Manual Fundamentals of Laparoscopy, Thoracoscopy, and GI Endoscopy. New York: Springer; 2006:467-495

[17] Tamm C, Scheidbach H, Hampe C, Schneider C, Köckerling F. Totally Extraperitoneal endoscopic inguinal hernia repair (TEP). Surgical Endoscopy. 2003;**17**(2):190-195

Chapter 8

Management of Obturator Hernia

Luigi Conti, Carmine Grassi, Filippo Banchini, Deborah Bonfili, Gaetano Maria Cattaneo, Edoardo Baldini and Patrizio Capelli

Abstract

The obturator hernia is a rare pelvic hernia that often presents with symptoms of bowel obstruction. Obturator hernia corresponds to 0.5–1.4% of all abdominal hernias. Entrapment of an intestinal segment within the obturator orifice, most often the ileum, less frequently Meckel's diverticulum or omentum, can cause intestinal obstruction. The non-specific presenting symptoms make the diagnosis of this condition often unclear. Females are 6–9 times more likely than men to be subject to the pathology, mostly occurring in a multiparous, emaciated, elderly woman so it is also called "the little old lady's hernia." Risk factors such as chronic constipation, chronic obstructive pulmonary disease, ascites, kyphoscoliosis, and multiparty, can predispose patients to herniation. A sign of inconstant presentation may be the presence of a palpable mass or pain radiating from the inner thigh and knee—known as Howship–Romberg sign—but it could be misleading when confused with symptoms of gonarthrosis or lumbar vertebral disc pathology. CT scan of the abdomen and pelvis has been found to be the gold standard for preoperative diagnosis because of its superior sensitivity and accuracy with respect to other radiological exams. The only possible treatment for this pathology is surgery, and management depends on early diagnosis.

Keywords: obturator hernia, old's lady hernia, bowel occlusion, laparoscopy, Howship–Romberg sign

1. Introduction

1.1 Anatomy and embryogenesis

An obturator hernia (OH) is the protrusion of either an intraperitoneal or an extraperitoneal organ or tissue through the obturator canal [1]. The development of ossification of the ischium and pubis occurs between the 4th and 5th months of gestation, so perhaps it can be assumed that potential bone formation to fill the obturator foramen stops during this period. For anatomical purposes, the obturator foramen is a lacuna, and the obturator canal is the true foramen [2]. The obturator hole is an orifice located in the lower half of the iliac bone, below the acetabulum, limited by the pubis and the ischium (**Figure 1**). This orifice is almost completely blocked by the obturator membrane, a fibrous membrane in continuity with the periosteum of the

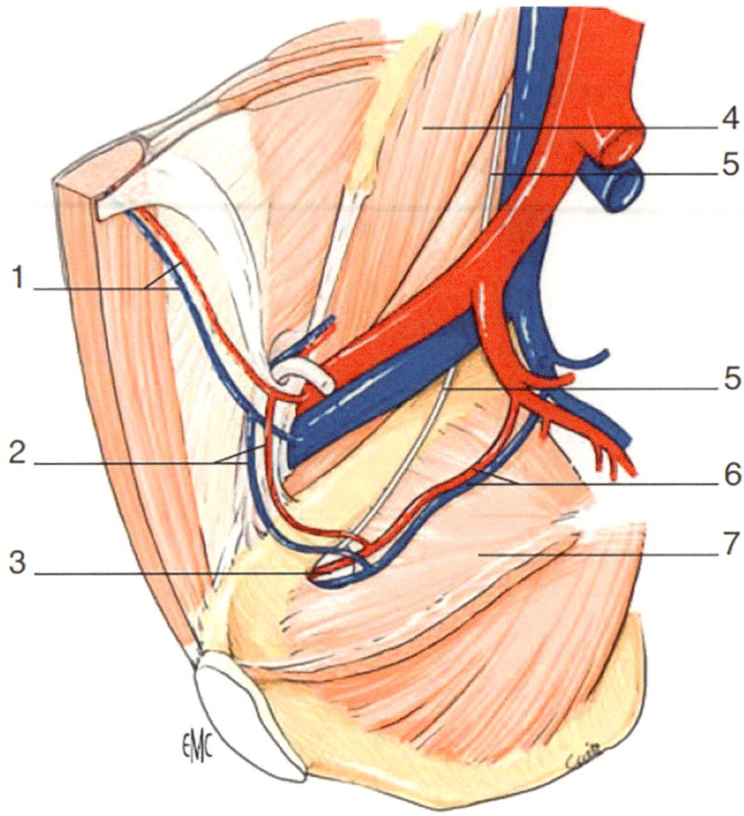

Figure 1.
Endopelvic view of the obturatory canal. 1: superficial epigastric vessels; 2: anastomosis between epigastric and obturator vessels; 3: obturator foramen; 4: ileo-psoas muscle; 5: obturator nerve; 6: obturator vessels; 7: internal obturator muscle. with permission from Ref. [3].

margins of the foramen itself. This membrane consists of two layers and is covered by the internal and external obturator muscles that latch on it and the bone margin (**Figure 2**) [2].

The obturator membrane does not cover the entire foramen: upwards it leaves a passage between its upper edge and the lower border of the horizontal branch of the pubis. This path is the obturator canal: an osteo-fibrous duct 2–3 cm long, directed obliquely from the inside out, which connects the pelvic cavity with the pre-obturator space of the thigh, between the external obturator muscle dorsally and muscles long adductor, comb, ileo-psoas ventrally. Its upper wall is the lower face of the horizontal branch of the pubis and as a floor, the obturator membrane, reinforced by an internal ligament. The canal is crossed by the obturator artery, vein and nerve. The obturator canal inwards is closed by the peritoneum, which may have a dimple at this level (obturator dimple) (**Figure 1**), enough to explain the possibility of obturator hernias, which occur in the upper part of the inner thigh region [5]. The canal offers a passage to the obturator peduncle, where the nerve is located above the artery and vein, and which contains a portion of adipose tissue. The obturator nerve, originating from L2, L3 and L4, divides into two branches at the emergence of the obturator canal. The ventral branch innervates the pectinate and the adductors muscles and supplies sensory branches to the medial face of the thigh; the dorsal branch also innervates the

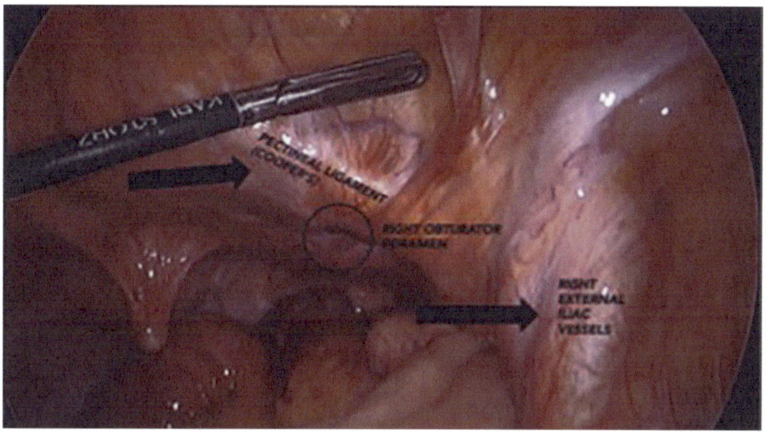

Figure 2.
In vivo anatomy of the right obturator foramen. (with permission from Ref. [4]).

adductors and ends at the knee joint level. This anatomical arrangement explains the Howship–Romberg sign: in case of compression of the obturator nerve by a strangulated hernia, it occurs obturator neuralgia exacerbated by extension, abduction and internal rotation of the thigh, resolved by flexion [6].

The obturator artery originates from the internal iliac artery and it is divided into two branches, medial and lateral, forming a circle around the perimeter of the obturator foramen, in the thickness of its musculoaponeurotic operculum.

There is an anastomosis between the obturator artery and inferior or superficial epigastric artery which crosses the horizontal branch of the pubis. There may be an aberrant obturator artery that can originate from the superficial epigastric artery or the external iliac artery. These arteries are accompanied by satellite veins. This vascular circle has been called "corona mortis", due to the high risk of bleeding. An anatomic variant has also been reported in which a pubic branch of the epigastric artery descending into the obturator foramen can replace the obturator artery, and a larger pubic vein draining into the iliac vein may replace the obturator vein.

2. Etiology

Arnaud de Ronsil in 1724 first described the obturator hernia, and then Henry Obre first successfully repaired it in 1851 [7].

Three anatomic stages in the formation of obturator hernia have been described. The first stage is the entrance of the pre-peritoneal fat tissue into the pelvic orifice of the obturator canal, forming a pilot fat plug. During the second stage, a peritoneal dimple develops through the canal and progresses to the formation of a peritoneal sac. The third stage consists of the onset of symptoms resulting from the herniation of the viscera into this sac [7, 8]. The formation of obturator hernia is favored by weight loss which involves the disappearance of the adipose tissue at the level of the obturator canal. This hernia is mainly formed in the elderly and thin women. In the beginning, the penetration of the extra-peritoneal tissue into the sub-pubic canal, then there is the formation of a dimple at the level of the peritoneum that covers it. Finally, a sac is formed with the risk of intestinal loops being inserted and their throttling due to the stiffness of the margins of the orifice. The sac can externalize directly through the exopelvic orifice of the canal, between the external obturator and pectineus muscles. However, it can also pass through the external obturator muscle or even fit between the two obturator muscles. The contents of the sac are usually the small intestine, more seldom an annex or ovary, bladder, appendix or epiploon. The narrowness of the orifice favors strangulation.

3. Clinical presentation

Obturator hernia is a rare pelvic hernia, accounting for the 0.5–1.4% of all hernias (**Table 1**) [9] that frequently causes bowel obstruction; the hernia passes through the obturator canal, bounded above by the obturator groove of the pubic bone, and below by the obturator membrane (**Figures 3** and **4**). The obturator canal is usually filled with fat and allows no space for hernia [3]. The fat disappears in patients who have had massive weight loss or are very thin indeed it is observed in elderly emaciated and multiparous women, so it's also called "little old's lady hernia" [10]. Right-sided OH is commoner than the left in the ratio of 2:1, as the left obturator foramen may be covered by the sigmoid colon [11], although an incidence of 6% bilateral hernias have been reported [12]. The hernia sac usually contains small bowel, rarely appendix, colon, Meckel diverticulum, or omentum [13]. A prompt diagnosis and treatment could avoid complications such as necrosis of the intestine that increases morbidity and mortality. Signs such as Howship–Romberg and Hannington–Kiff are aspecific and they should be associated with a CT-scan which is clearly the choice radiological exam. Symptoms such as the pain radiating from the inner parts of the thigh, the knee, or the hip could be confused with the dorso-lumbar intervertebral disc pathology or gonarthrosis [14, 15].

Obturator hernia poses a diagnostic challenge and the signs and symptoms are often aspecific, which makes a preoperative diagnosis difficult. Obturator hernia should be included in the differential diagnosis of intestinal obstruction of unknown origin, especially in emaciated elderly women with chronic disease. The almost exclusive incidence of obturatory hernia in women can be explained by the greater extension of the obturator foramen and from the different obliquity of the pelvis that exposes it to a direct action of abdominal pressure in women. More frequent symptoms are due to an intestinal obstruction like abdominal pain, distension, nausea, vomiting and constipation [16]. They may also have recurrent attacks of intestinal obstruction in the past with or without a palpable mass in the groin. On

Hernia type	Percentage of presentation
Inguinal	75%
Incisional	10–15%
Femural	5–10%
Umbilical	—
Spigelian (at linea semilunaris)	—
Epigastric (linea alba)	—
Obturator	0.5–1.6%

Table 1.
The frequency of presentation in the general population of the types of abdominal wall hernia.

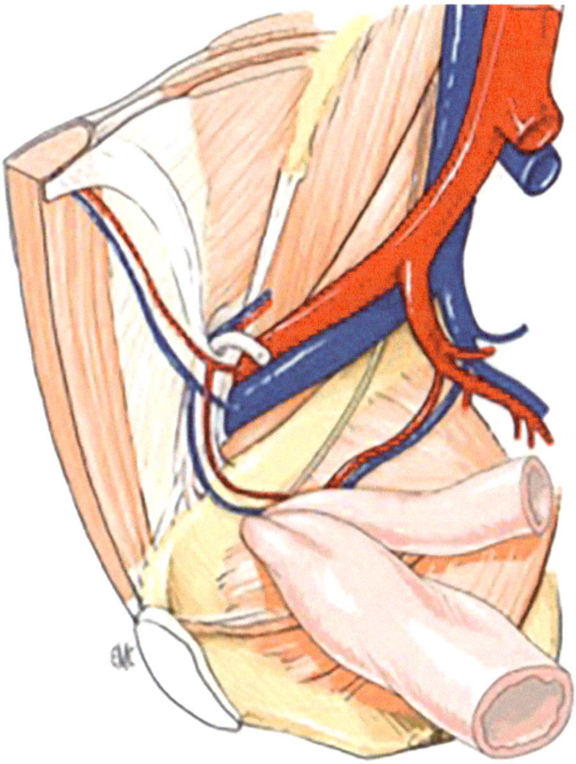

Figure 3.
Depiction of strangulated obturator hernia. (with permission from Ref. [3]).

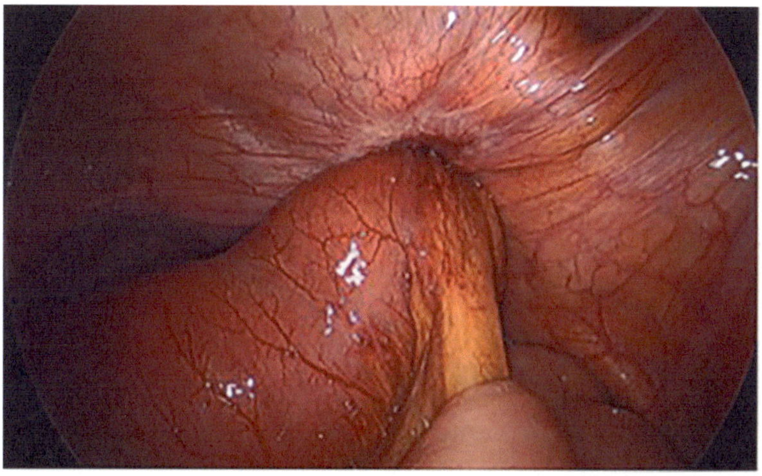

Figure 4.
Intraoperative findings: the small intestine is incarcerated in the obturator foramen. (with the permission from Ref. [4].

physical examination, it may be evident the Howship–Romberg sign: in case of compression of the obturatory nerve by a strangulated hernia, it occurs an obturator neuralgia exacerbated by extension, abduction and internal rotation of the thigh, resolved by flexion. It is considered pathognomonic and presents in 15–50% of cases. The Hannington–Kiff sign (absent adductor reflex and an intact patellar reflex) is reported as more specific [17]. It would be necessary to perform a computed tomography (CT) to make a diagnosis. The CT has an accuracy of 90% [18]. An emergency exploratory laparotomy is fundamental in patients presenting with an acute abdomen.

4. Diagnosis

Abdominal plain radiograph shows aspecific signs of intestinal obstruction and very rarely may show a gas shadow in the area of obturator foramen, therefore, it is not an informative exam [19].

Herniography with the intraperitoneal injection of contrast material under local anesthesia was reported to be useful for demonstrating the hernial sac but it is not a reproducible examination in emergency conditions because it can be done only in elective cases [20].

Ultrasonography (US) is a noninvasive, cheap, and easily available diagnostic tool that can be used to diagnose OH accurately, especially in the emergency setup when patients present with the acute abdomen of uncertain cause, hence allowing early operative treatment. Using a high-frequency probe, the examiner could detect a hypoechoic mass corresponding to the dilated and edematous segment of the intestine posterior to the pectineus muscle [21]. The major advantages of US are that it is a non-invasive and allows for comparison with the asymptomatic side. Limiting factors are dependence on examiner experience (who may at times miss the diagnosis by not scanning the femoral region or may not recognize the hernia as it is small and found deep within the pelvic musculature) and the relatively long learning curve. Also, too much pressure on the transducer can reduce the sensitivity of detection of hernias [22].

Barium enema fluoroscopy can demonstrate a hank of intestinal loops but is very time-consuming and not feasible in cases of acute abdomen. Also, retained barium in the bowel loop may increase the risk of subsequent complications, hence it is not routinely advocated [23].

Magnetic resonance is a comparable method to CT scan for diagnosis but is not always available in urgency or in most cases of obturator hernia presentation [24].

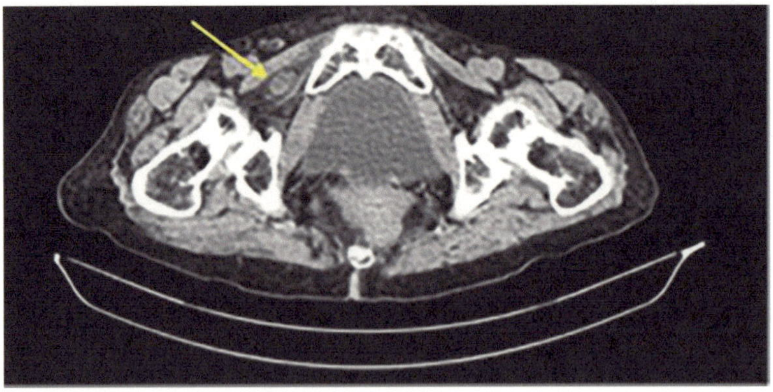

Figure 5.
CT scan, coronal: the arrow identifies the right obturator hernia sac; the small intestine is dilated. (with permission from Ref. [4].

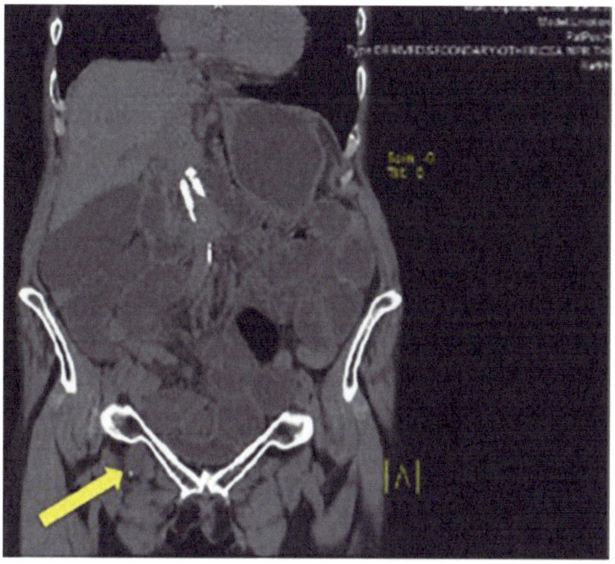

Figure 6.
CT scan transverse section. (with permission from Ref. [4]).

CT scan (**Figure 5**) is more sensitive and specific, showing a mass-like lesion between the obturator externus and pectineus muscles (**Figure 6**), it is useful to shorten the lapse of time from presentation to appropriate diagnosis and spontaneously subjecting a patient to definitive surgery, and thus also giving a choice in the surgical approach required [14].

5. Treatment

Once the diagnosis is obtained or in the diagnostic suspicion of obturator hernia, therapy is exclusively surgical: in the presence of signs of intestinal obstruction or incarceration, surgical exploration is mandatory. The manual reduction of an incarcerated obturator hernia has been described in cases of patients considered unfit for surgery, but two aspects must be considered: the early recurrence and the impossibility to explore the incarcerated viscera in case of possible evolution to gangrene or bowel infarction. If the incarcerated obturator hernia is not treated, it can be fatal and in any case, should always be repaired both in case of urgency and in case of non-acute symptomatology attributable to the hernia; it should be remembered that symptoms may persist and then result in incarceration. The current trend is to repair the obturatory foramen with the use of prostheses primarily made of polypropylene; however, if the orifice is less than 1 cm, the approach could also consist of direct repair. Currently, there is no consensus on the repair technique but it is all based on the surgeon's experience and preference. The different feasible surgical approaches are intraabdominal, inguinal extraperitoneal, obturator or crural, Cheatle–Henry retropubic and laparoscopic approach [24–27].

5.1 Intra-abdominal approach

In an emergency set-up usually, a midline incision by laparotomy is required to allow a wider exposure of the obturator ring, the pelvic floor and the lower abdomen, especially in the case of gangrenous bowel resection. Uncoiling the bowel discovers the dilated tract at the border with the strangulated one, usually with a lateral clamping: it is necessary to gently pull the bowel to reduce it in the abdomen avoiding rupture that would lead to septic contamination. The bowel is treated as in all cases of strangulation, preserving or resecting it depending on the degree of intestinal wall perfusion. Suturing the small orifice can be done with several techniques: simple direct closure with several stitches, two layers closure of peritoneum (**Figure 7**). For large defect: patching and plugging the canal with rib cartilage, peritoneal patch, periosteal patch, pectineal or adductor longus muscle flap with external oblique aponeurosis, greater omentum, round ligament, uterine fundus, ovary, urinary bladder wall, ox fascia, tantalum gauze, teflon cloth, marlex mesh, oxidized cellulose gauze (oxycel), polytetrafluoroethylene (PTFE), polypropylene mesh, Kugel patch, permacol patch plug [19] of mersilene, rolled up marlex mesh as a "cigar roll" plug and titanium alloy staples without mesh [24–28].

5.2 Laparoscopic approach

The laparoscopic approach, both–trans-abdominal pre-peritoneal (TAPP) or total extraperitoneal (TEP) [29], is feasible in expert settings: the position of the trocars,

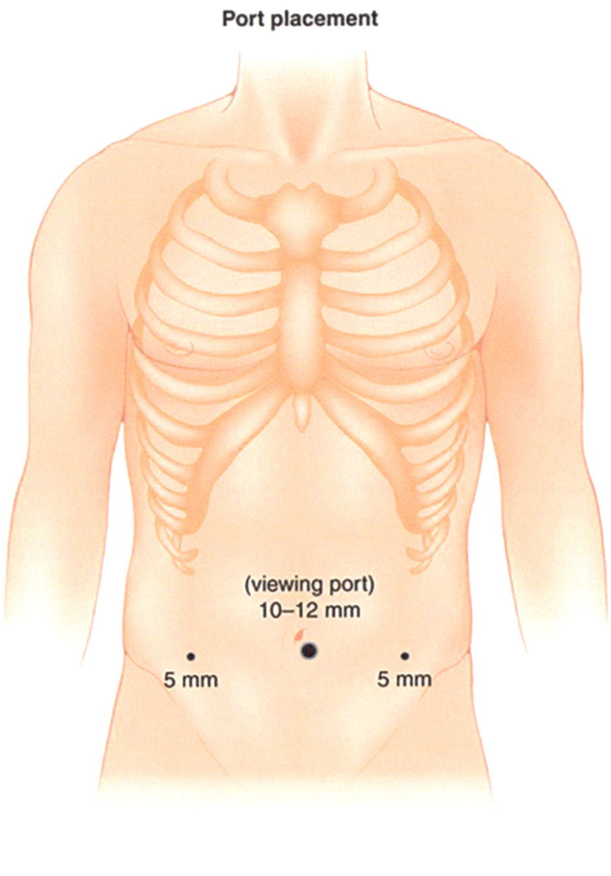

Figure 7.
Trocars placement in obturator hernia laparoscopic repair.

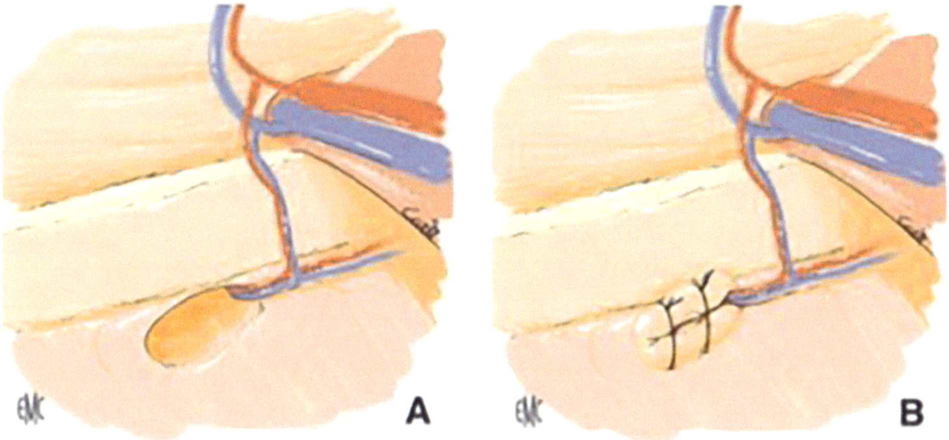

Figure 8.
The obturator orifice (A) is repaired with direct intra-abdominal suture (B). (with permission from Ref. [3]).

patient and operators is similar to that of the TAPP and TEP repair for inguinal hernia (**Figure 8**) [30–32]. Placement of a double-layer prosthesis is not recommended in the same manner as in abdominal wall hernias because the peripheral anchorage is not safe due to the presence of vascular and nerve structures. It is necessary to proceed as in TAPP repair for inguinal hernia: the peritoneum is dissected above the inguinal dimples, the dissection is conducted lower than the orifice of the obturator canal, the sac is reduced in the abdomen, and the prosthesis is placed in the extraperitoneal space with an overlap of at least 3–4 cm. The peritoneum is sutured above the prosthesis.

5.3 Inguinal approach

The procedure is similar to the Stoppa inguinal hernia repair. Through a median or Pfannenstiel incision, the Retzius' space is dissected, posterior to the pubic symphysis, the dissection is extended laterally to the antero-superior iliac spine. The peritoneum is detached from the anterior abdominal wall and the epigastric vessels are left attached. Once the sac is reduced in the abdomen, it is possible to place a large prosthesis covering the inguinal, femoral and obturator region attached to the transverse and rectus abdominis muscles medially and on the pubic symphysis inferiorly.

5.4 Femoral approach

A 10-cm vertical incision is made on the medial margin of the femoral triangle medial to the femoral vessels and adductor muscles, passed by blunt dissection between the pectinate and middle adductor muscles. The sac can be resected and the orifice closed with a plug or direct suture. This approach is not the recommended one [3].

Other possible approaches can be performed via combined abdomino-crural, cruro-obturator, inguino-obturator, subcrural intraperitoneal [33–35]. The obturator dimple can be repaired using a direct suture (**Figure 9**), with a recurrence rate lower than 3%, or use a resorbable mesh or plug [36, 37]. Patches of peritoneum or omentum may be used in cases of small orifices [38, 39].

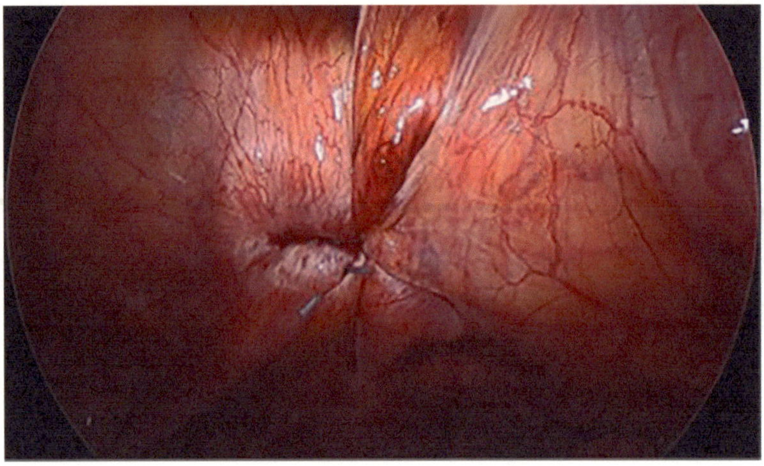

Figure 9.
Primary laparoscopic repair by using non-absorbable suture. (with permission from Ref. [4]).

6. Conclusion

Due to its rarity of presentation obturator hernia presents a diagnostic challenge and should be included in the differential diagnosis of intestinal obstruction of unknown origin, especially in emaciated elderly women with chronic disease; a prompt suspect based on aspecific symptoms is crucial for the diagnosis. CT scan has a major sensitivity than other radiological exams. Late diagnosis of obturator hernia can lead to ischemia and bowel necrosis with bowel perforation and then localized or generalized peritonitis as a life-threatening condition. Postoperative complications have been reported in 11.6% of patients as pneumonia, sepsis, wound infection [40, 41] and mesh migration which may be prevented with metal anchors [42, 43]. The resultant morbidity and mortality rates are around 38% and 12–70%, respectively. Surgical management depends on early diagnosis and it is the only possible treatment for this pathology [4].

Acknowledgements

This work has been funded by AUSL Piacenza, Unit of Research and Quality.

Dr. Conti conceived the book chapter; Dr. Conti and Dr. Bonfili wrote the chapter and processed the images. Dr. Baldini and Dr. Conti performed the surgery. Dr. Cattaneo, Dr. Grassi, Dr. Banchini and Dr. Capelli reviewed the literature. All authors reviewed and approved the chapter.

Conflict of interest

The authors declare no conflict of interest.

Notes/thanks/other declarations

We would like to thank the physicians of the Acute Care Surgery team of AUSL Piacenza, Dr. Sonia Agrusti, Dr. Mauro Filosa, Dr. Luigi Percalli, Dr. Gabriele Regina,

Dr. Giandomenico Arzu, Dr. Giancarlo Giannone and Dr. Antonio Caizzone for their contributions and expertise in the field of hernia surgery.

We would also like to thank the editor Elsevier-Masson, SAS Paris, for the kind permission to reuse the iconography from the EMC Surgical techniques book.

Author details

Luigi Conti[1*], Carmine Grassi[1], Filippo Banchini[2], Deborah Bonfili[3], Gaetano Maria Cattaneo[1], Edoardo Baldini[4] and Patrizio Capelli[2]

1 Acute Care Surgery Unit, Department of Surgery, AUSL Piacenza, Italy

2 General, Vascular and Thoracic Surgery Unit, Department of Surgery, AUSL Piacenza, Italy

3 Department of Medicine and Surgery, University Hospital of Parma, Italy

4 General Surgery Unit, ASST Melegnano-Martesana, Melzo (Milan), Italy

*Address all correspondence to: dr.luigiconti@gmail.com

IntechOpen

© 2022 The Author(s). Licensee IntechOpen. This chapter is distributed under the terms of the Creative Commons Attribution License (http://creativecommons.org/licenses/by/3.0), which permits unrestricted use, distribution, and reproduction in any medium, provided the original work is properly cited.

References

[1] Lien W-C. Obturator Hernia: The "little old Lady's Hernia". Journal of Medical Ultrasound. 2014;**22**:96-98

[2] Skandalakis LJ, Androulakis J, Colborn GL, Skandalakis JE. Obturator hernia: Embryology, anatomy, and surgical applications. The Surgical Clinics of North America. 2000;**80**(1):71-84

[3] Pélissier E, Ngo P, Armstrong O. Trattamento chirurgico delle ernie otturatorie. In: Tecniche Chirurgiche – Abdominal. Paris: EMC, Elsevier Masson SAS; 2010. pp. 40-155

[4] Conti L, Baldini E, Capelli P, Capelli C. Bowel obstruction in obturator hernia: A challenging diagnosis. International Journal of Surgery Case Reports. 2018;**42**:154-157

[5] Fumagalli C. Normal human anatomy. Piccin Ed Padova. 1982;**1**:583

[6] Hsu CH, Wang CC, Jeng LB, Chen MF. Obturator hernia: A report of eight cases. The American Surgeon. 1993;**59**:709-711

[7] Tsai M-T, Jiann-Ming W, Lien W-C, Hernia O. The "little old Lady's Hernia". Journal of Medical Ultrasound. 2014;**2**(22):96-98

[8] Haraguchi M, Matsuo S, Kanetaka K, et al. Obturator hernia in an ageing society. Annals of the Academy of Medicine, Singapore. 2007;**36**:413-415

[9] Rodríguez-Hermosa JI, Codina-Cazador A, Maroto-Genover A, et al. Obturator hernia: Clinical analysis of 16 cases and algorithm for its diagnosis and treatment. Hernia. 2008;**12**:289-297

[10] Losanoff JE, Richman BW, Jones JW. Obturator hernia. Journal of the American College of Surgeons. 2002;**194**:657-663

[11] Granite G, Meshida K, Wind G. Frequency and clinical review of the aberrant obturator artery: A cadaveric study. Diagnostics (Basel). 2020;**10**(8): 546

[12] Anagnostopoulou S, Kostopanagiotou G, Paraskeuopoulos T, Chantzi C, Lolis E, Saranteas T. Anatomic variations of the obturator nerve in the inguinal region: Implications in conventional and ultrasound regional anesthesia techniques. Regional Anesthesia and Pain Medicine. 2009;**34**(1):33-39

[13] Rusu MC, Cergan R, Motoc AG, Folescu R, Pop E. Anatomical considerations on the corona mortis. Surgical and Radiologic Anatomy. 2010;**32**(1):17-24

[14] Drewes PG, Marinis SI, Schaffer JI, Boreham MK, Corton MM. Vascular anatomy over the superior pubic rami in female cadavers. American Journal of Obstetrics and Gynecology. 2005;**193**(6):2165-2168

[15] Park J. Obturator hernia: Clinical analysis of 11 patients and review of the literature. Medicine (Baltimore). 2020;**99**(34):e21701

[16] Mandarry MT, Zeng S-B, Wei Z-Q, Zhang C, Wang Z-W. Obturator hernia - a condition seldom thought of and hence seldom sought. International Journal of Colorectal Disease. 2012;**27**:133-141

[17] Yokoyama Y, Yamaguchi A, Isogai M, Hori A, Kaneoka Y. Thirty-six cases of obturator hernia: Does computed tomography contribute to postoperative

outcome? World Journal of Surgery. 1999;**23**(2):214-217

[18] Terado R, Ito S, Kidogawa H, Kidogawa H, Kashima K, Ooe H. Obturator hernia: The usefulness of emergent computed tomography for early diagnosis. The Journal of Emergency Medicine. 1999;**17**(5):883-886

[19] Young C, Bourne R, Gopalswamy S. Permacol patch repair for obstructed obturator hernia: A case report and review of literature. The Internet Journal of Surgery. 2009;**20**(2)

[20] Avaro JP, Biance N, Savoie PH, Peycru T, Pauleau G, Richez P, et al. Incarcerated obturator hernia: Early diagnostic using helical computed tomography. Hernia. 2008;**12**(2008): 199-200

[21] Igari K, Ochiai T, Aihara A, Kumagai Y, Iida M, Yamazaki S. Clinical presentation of obturator hernia and review of the literature. Hernia. 2010;**14**:409-413

[22] Dundamadappa SK, Tsou IYY, Goh JSK. Clinics in diagnostic imaging. Singapore Medical Journal. 2006;**47**(107):89-95

[23] Nakayama T, Kobayashi S, Shiraishi K, Nishiumi T, Mori S, Isobe K, et al. Diagnosis and treatment of obturator hernia. The Keio Journal of Medicine. 2002;**51**:129-132

[24] Mercado M, Diab J, Loi K. A delayed diagnosis of obturator hernia hoodwinked by previous laparoscopic inguinal hernia repair. Journal of Surgical Case Reports. 2021;**9**

[25] Lobo DN, Clarke DJ, Barlow AP. Obturator hernia: A new technique for repair. Journal of the Royal College of Surgeons of Edinburgh. 1998;**43**:33-33

[26] Murai S, Akatsu T, Yabe N, Inoue Y, Akatsu Y, Kitagawa Y. Impacted obturator hernia treated successfully with a kugel repair: Report of two cases. Surgery Today. 2009;**39**(2009):821-824

[27] Martínez Insua C, Costa Pereira JM, Cardoso de Oliveira M. Obturator hernia: The plug technique. Hernia. 2001;**5**:161-116

[28] De Leo S, Gullà N, Patriti A, Bufalari A, Capitanucci L, Ciaccio V, et al. Obturator hernia: A new device in mesh repair. Hernia. 2000;**4**(200):155-158

[29] Chang SS, Shan YS, Lin YJ, Tai YS, Lin PW. A review of obturator hernia and a proposed algorithm for its diagnosis and treatment. World Journal of Surgery. 2005;**29**:450-454

[30] Bjork KJ, Mucha P Jr, Calull DR. Obturator hernia. Surgery, Gynecology & Obstetrics. 1988;**167**(3):217-222

[31] Mantoo SK, Mak K, Tan TJ. Obturator hernia: Diagnosis and treatment in the modern era. Singapore Medical Journal. 2009;**50**(9):866-870

[32] Liao CF, Liu CC, Chuang CH, Hsu KC. Obturator hernia: Adiagnostic challenge of small bowel obstruction. The American Journal of the Medical Sciences. 2010;**339**:92-94

[33] Shapiro K, Patel S, Choy C, Chaudry G, Khalil S, Ferzli G. Totally extraperitoneal repair of obturator hernia. Surgical Endoscopy. 2004;**18**(6):954-956

[34] Dorai Thambi CR. Obturator hernia—Review of three cases. Singapore Medical Journal. 1988;**29**(2):179-181

[35] Pandey R, Maqbool A, Jayachandran N. Obturator hernia:

A diagnostic challenge. Hernia. 2009;**13**:97-99

[36] Kulkarni SR, Punamiya AR, Naniwadekar RG, Janugade HB, Tejas D, Chotai T, et al. Obturator hernia: A diagnostic challenge. International Journal of Surgery Case Reports. 2013;**4**(7):606-608

[37] Mahendran B, Lopez PP. Obturator Hernia. [Updated 2021 Jul 26]. In: StatPearls [Internet]. Treasure Island (FL): StatPearls Publishing; 2021

[38] Chitrambalam TG, Christopher PJ, Sundaraj J, Selvamuthukumaran S. Diagnostic difficulties in obturator hernia: A rare case presentation and review of literature. BML Case Reports. 2020;**13**(9):e235644

[39] Elena M-F, Stephanie G-B, Fernando L-M, Roberto M-O, Alfredo M-L, Salvador L. Computed tomographic diagnosis of obturator hernia and its surgical management: A case series. International Journal of Surgery. 2007;**5**(3):139-142

[40] Glicklich M, Eliasoph J. Incarcerated obturator hernia: Case diagnosed at barium enema fluoroscopy. Radiology. 1989;**172**:51-52

[41] Marchal F, Parent S, Tortuyaux JM, Bresler L, Boissel P, Regent D. Obturator hernias—Report of seven cases. Hernia. 1997;**1**:23-26

[42] Zhang H, Cong JC, Chen CS. Ileum perforation due to delayed operation in obturator hernia: A case report and review of literatures. World Journal of Gastroenterology. 2010;**16**:126-130

[43] Borchert D, Kumar B, Dennis R, Alberts J. Mesh migration following obturator hernia repair presenting as a bezoar inducing small intestinal obstruction. Hernia. 2008;**12**(2008):83-85

Chapter 9

Hybrid: Evolving Techniques in Laparoscopic Ventral Hernia Mesh Repair

Wasim Dar, Uday Muddebihal and Uliargoli Vasudeva Rao

Abstract

Laparoscopic repair is now the treatment of choice for most cases of ventral/incisional hernia. It is superior to open repair. Although the technique has undergone many refinements, there is no standard technique for difficult or complicated hernias. In cases with difficult hernias, combined open/laparoscopic hybrid techniques to avoid dissection of large subcutaneous flaps benefit the patients. It has been reported that hybrid methods are effective for treating cases of ventral hernias involving a large orifice. The techniques used and proposed by us are - (1) laparoscopic adhesiolysis, open sac excision with closure of defect and laparoscopic mesh placement, (2) laparoscopic adhesiolysis, omphalectomy with closure of defect and laparoscopic mesh placement and (3) open adhesiolysis, sac excision with closure of defect and laparoscopic mesh placement Laparoscopic Ventral Hernia Hybrid Mesh Repair (LVHHMR) is safe and feasible approach for complicated/difficult ventral hernias.

Keywords: composite mesh, hybrid techniques, laparoscopic ventral hernia mesh repair

1. Introduction

Hernia is the protrusion of viscus or part of viscus through a weakness/defect in anterior abdominal wall. It can be seen in all age groups and in either of the sexes. It is a common surgical condition.

The surgical description and treatments of hernia dates to most of the ancient civilisations. One of the earliest documentations appeared in 1500 BC in Epytian papyrus of Ebers. The repair of hernia went through many changes during 15th to 20th centuries. Surgical meshes for repair of hernias have been used since 1891.

In 1979, P. Fletcher performed the first laparoscopic hernia surgery.

Laparoscopic ventral hernia repair is superior to open technique and now a first option for most of the cases [1]. Over the past four decades this procedure has undergone many changes, however, there is no gold standard technique for difficult or complicated hernias.

There are lots of debate and research going on to standardize the technique of laparoscopic ventral hernia repair, including the ideal mesh, closure of defect and fixation methods [2].

IntechOpen

One of the areas of non-consensus, over the period was regarding the closure of the defect. Many centers did not close the hernia defect, but directly placed a mesh and fixed it. However, now there is huge data available to support the fact that primary closure of the hernial defect allows better reinforcement of the wall and by reducing the dead space, it decreases the chances of seroma formation [3].

It is challenging to deal with difficult hernias, and hence patient undergoes conventional open repair with dissection of large subcutaneous flaps and post-operative morbidity. Recent studies have shown that hybrid techniques involving both open and laparoscopic methods benefit the patients [4]. It's been reported that Hybrid methods are effective for treating cases of ventral hernias involving a large orifice [5].

2. Types of hernia

A. Based on the cause

a. Congenital – birth defects

b. Acquired - develop later in life

B. Based on the site [6]–

1. Groin hernias

a. Inguinal hernias – (70–75% of all abdominal hernias) Abdominal contents protrude into the groin through the inguinal canal.

b. Femoral hernias – (6–18% of all abdominal hernias) Abdominal contents protrude into the groin through the femoral triangle

2. Ventral hernias – These hernias can be

a. Umbilical

b. Paraumbilical

c. Epigastric

d. Spigelian

e. Incisional

3. Hiatus hernia – A part of stomach or intestine protrude into the chest via the diaphragm

C. Based on clinical presentation

1. Reducible

2. Irreducible

3. Obstructed

4. Strangulated

3. Ventral hernias

The most common types of ventral hernias are umbilical, paraumbilical and incisional hernias. The acquired risk factors for such hernias are – Chronic cough, constipation, heavy weightlifting, trauma, obesity, pregnancy, and prior surgery.

Clinical diagnosis is made by proper history of lump, duration, pain, reducibility, and obstruction. Including, complete physical examination involving all hernial orifices, cough impulse and tenderness. Imaging such as Ultrasound, CT and MRI are done to confirm the clinical diagnosis and to know the features of hernia such as site, size, number, and contents.

4. Treatment

A hernia does not go away without surgery. The closure of hernial defect with the use of mesh has been widely accepted.

Techniques of ventral hernia repair

A. Open technique

B. Laparoscopic technique (LVHR)

C. Hybrid techniques (LVHHMR)

In most of the patients with small hernial defects and uncomplicated clinical presentation, laparoscopic approach for repair and mesh placement is now the preferred method of management [7, 8].

Open approach for large, multiple defects and complicated hernias is used and accepted. The morbidity associated with open repair are dissection of large subcutaneous flaps, multiple drain placements, delayed post-operative recovery, more chances of infection and recurrence [9]. To avoid such complications a combination of laparoscopic and open techniques is being reported.

It has been established that to avoid seroma formation and recurrence of hernia, the defect must be closed [10]. Patients that undergo laparoscopic hernia mesh have comparatively lesser complications like decreased operative time, no drains, decreased post-operative pain, early discharge and getting back to work. Avoids complications of open repair [11, 12].

In hybrid technique, various combinations of steps of open and laparoscopic hernia repair are used. The basic principle involves hernia sac excision, closure of all the defects and removal of necrotic skin (if applicable). Here a composite mesh is always used laparoscopically.

Research show that the hybrid technique, when used in recurrent difficult incisional hernias is safe [13]. Some reports also suggest that hybrid techniques should be used in hernia with difficult defects, hernias with necrotic skin, irreducible hernias, obese patients with difficult incisional hernias, lateral incisional hernias [14] and parastomal hernias [15].

5. How we do it?

We have been doing Laparoscopic Ventral Hernia Hybrid Technique Mesh Repair (LVHHMR) since 2014.

All patients presenting with complicated ventral hernia of defect diameter of up to 8 cms and fit for surgery undergo LVHHMR. The common complications that the patients present with are, large defects, obstructed hernia with bowel contents, irreducible hernia with necrotic umbilical skin and multiple defects.

Patients unfit for general anesthesia, BMI > 35 kg/m2, hernia defects more than 8 cms, pregnancy and contaminated abdominal cavity do not undergo such repair.

The routine clinical diagnosis supported with abdominal ultrasound is done in all the patients. Pre anesthesia evaluation and informed written consent is taken before the surgery. Standardized procedure, involving patient in supine position and general anesthesia with endotracheal intubation is done in all the patients.

Palmers point approach is used to create pneumoperitoneum (2 cms below left subcostal margin in mid-clavicular line) [16]. Alternatively, optical port entry is also used in some patients.

Under vision two further ports are introduced, one 10 mm port in epigastric region (for 30° laparoscope) and another 5 mm port in the right flank at the level of umbilicus. Alternatively, all the three ports are placed in the left flank.

6. The LVHHMR techniques include

1. Laparoscopic adhesiolysis, open sac excision with closure of defect and a laparoscopic mesh placement

2. Laparoscopic adhesiolysis, omphalectomy with closure of defect and laparoscopic mesh placement.

3. Open adhesiolysis, sac excision with closure of defect and laparoscopic mesh placement.

4. Laparoscopic adhesiolysis, open sac excision with closure of defect and a laparoscopic mesh placement –

Used in patients with large hernial sac. Harmonic shears or Bi-polar is used for laparoscopic adhesiolysis. Contents of hernia sac are reduced. A small circum-umbilical incision is taken, and complete hernia sac is excised. Closure of the defect with interrupted prolene sutures and skin closed.

1. Laparoscopic adhesiolysis, omphalectomy with closure of defect and laparoscopic mesh placement –

This is done in patients with large sac, multiple defects, and necrotic umbilical skin. Laparoscopic adhesiolysis is done and contents reduced. Abdomen desufflated and omphalectomy is done. Hernia sac is then excised, and the defect closed with interrupted prolene sutures and skin closed.

2. Open adhesiolysis, sac excision with closure of defect and laparoscopic mesh placement –

This is done in patients with large hernia sac, small defect, and obstructed bowel. Diagnostic laparoscopy is performed. Abdomen desufflated and infra umbilical incision is taken. Open adhesiolysis is done. Hernia sac is excised, and the defect is closed with interrupted prolene sutures and skin closed.

7. Meshes used

In laparoscopic and hybrid procedures the mesh is placed intraabdominally, and in direct contact with bowel and omentum. The accepted meshes are composite with partial absorbable properties and with collagen layers. The mesh sizes used are 15 x 15 cms circular (20), 15 x 20 rectangular (25) and 20 x 20 cms circular (30). The size of the mesh must overlap the defect from all sides by 4–5 cms.

8. Mesh fixations

Prefixed sutures on the mesh are used to lift it up on the anterior abdominal wall. Trans fascial sutures along with absorbable tackers are used to anchor the mesh. Alternatively, in light weight meshes and in patients with BMI less than 30, only tackers are used to fix the mesh. There is consensus in method of using tackers to fix the mesh. Circumferential row of tackers at extreme periphery of the mesh and another around the margins of the hernia defect. This technique is called the double crown technique [17] and emphasis is given to the distance between each tack (about 2–3 cms).

9. Literature

Our study (Hybrid: Evolving techniques in laparoscopic ventral hernia mesh repair) published in journal of minimal access surgery July 2020, has similar results as compared to that of literature [18]. We have demonstrated various hybrid techniques and their post-operative outcome.

10. Conclusion

Laparoscopic Ventral Hernia Hybrid Technique Mesh Repair (LVHHMR) is safe and feasible approach for complicated/difficult ventral hernias. However, further larger studies are required to establish these methods as gold standard.

Author details

Wasim Dar*, Uday Muddebihal and Uliargoli Vasudeva Rao
Sri Krishna Sevasharama Hospital, Bangalore, India

*Address all correspondence to: wassimd@yahoo.com

IntechOpen

© 2022 The Author(s). Licensee IntechOpen. This chapter is distributed under the terms of the Creative Commons Attribution License (http://creativecommons.org/licenses/by/3.0), which permits unrestricted use, distribution, and reproduction in any medium, provided the original work is properly cited.

References

[1] LeBlanc KA. Current considerations in laparoscopic incisional and ventral herniorrhaphy. JSLS. 2000;**4**(2):131-139

[2] Dąbrowiecki S, Pierściński S, Wojciech S. The Glubran 2 glue for mesh fixation in Lichtenstein's hernia repair: A double-blind randomized study. Videosurgery Miniinv. 2012;**7**:96-104

[3] Pielaciński K, Szczepanik AB, Misiak A, Wróblewski T. Randomized clinical trial comparing inguinal hernia repair with Lichtenstein technique using non-absorbable or partially absorbable mesh. Preliminary report. Videosurgery Miniinv. 2011;**6**:190-206

[4] Stoikes N, Quasebarth M, Brunt LM. Hybrid ventral hernia repair: technique and results. Hernia. 2013;**17**(5):627-632

[5] Yoshikawa K, Shimada M, Kurita N, Sato H, et al. Hybrid technique for laparoscopic incisional ventral hernia repair combining laparoscopic primary closure and mesh repair. International Surgery. 2005;**90**(3 Suppl):S56-S62

[6] Baylón K, Rodríguez-Camarillo P, Elías-Zúñiga A, Díaz-Elizondo JA, Gilkerson R, Lozano K. Past, present and future of surgical meshes: A review. Membranes (Basel). 2017;**7**(3):47

[7] Raftopoulos I, Courcoulas AP. Outcome of laparoscopic ventral hernia repair in morbidly obese patients with a body mass indexes exceeding 35 kg/m2. Surgical Endoscopy. 2007;**21**:2293-2297

[8] Uranues S, Salehi B, Bergamaschi R. Adverse events, quality of life and recurrence rates after laparoscopic adhesiolysis and recurrent incisional hernia mesh repair in patients with previous failed repairs. Journal of the American College of Surgeons. 2008;**207**:663

[9] Gonzalez R, Mason E, Duncan T, Wilson R, Ramshaw BJ. Laparoscopic versus open umbilical hernia repair. JSLS: Journal of the Society of Laparoendoscopic Surgeons. 2003;**7**(4):323-328

[10] Beldi G, Wagner M, Bruegger LE, et al. Mesh shrinkage and pain in laparoscopic ventral hernia repair: a randomized clinical trial comparing suture versus tack mesh fixation. Surgical Endoscopy. 2011;**25**:749-755

[11] Malik AM. Laparoscopic versus open repair of para-umbilical hernia. Is it a good alternative? The Journal of the Pakistan Medical Association. 2015;**65**(8):865-868

[12] Colavita PD, Tsirline VB, Walters AL, Lincourt AE, Belyansky I, Heniford BT. Laparoscopic versus open hernia repair: Outcomes and sociodemographic utilization results from the nationwide inpatient sample. Surgical Endoscopy. 2013;**27**(1):109-117

[13] Griniatsos J, Yiannakopoulou E, Tsechpenakis A, Tsigris C, Diamantis T. A hybrid technique for recurrent incisional hernia repair. Surgical Laparoscopy, Endoscopy & Percutaneous Techniques. 2009;**19**(5):e177-e180

[14] Schwab R, Sahm J, Willms AG, "Video-Assisted Mini-Open Sublay (VAMOS): A Simple Hybrid Approach for Lateral Incisional Hernias" Frontiers in Surgery. 2018;**5**:29.

[15] Luo W, Wang Y, Duan X. Therapeutic effect of a new hybrid technique

which combined laparoscopic method and abdominal repair for parastomal hernia repair. Zhonghua Wai Ke Za Zhi. 2017;**55**(7):539-542

[16] Palmer R. Safety in laparoscopy. The Journal of Reproductive Medicine. 1974;**13**:1-5

[17] Carbajo MA, Martin del Olmo JC, Blanco JI, et al. Laparoscopic approach to incisional hernia. Surgical Endoscopy. 2003;**17**:118-122

[18] Wasim MD, Muddebihal UM, Rao UV. Hybrid: Evolving techniques in laparoscopic ventral hernia mesh repair. Journal of Minimal Access Surgery. 2020;**16**(3):224-228. DOI: 10.4103/jmas.JMAS_163_18

Chapter 10

Robotic Complex Abdominal Wall Reconstruction: The Evolution of Component Separation

Rodolfo J. Oviedo, Jeffrey Hodges, Joseph Nguyen-Lee, David Detz, Mary Oh, João Bombardelli, Anuj Shah, Atteeba Manzar and Alessandro Martinino

Abstract

From the first description of the component separation technique in the literature at the end of the twentieth century to the current state of complex abdominal wall reconstruction, this rapidly evolving field of General Surgery has advanced at an accelerated pace. With the advancement of technological breakthroughs that stem from the original open technique, endoscopic, laparoscopic, and more recently robotic approaches have been developed to facilitate complex abdominal wall reconstruction to restore the body's anatomy and physiology to functional levels. This chapter will give an overview of the historic progression of these advanced techniques and will illustrate the key steps for their safe and effective performance including the endoscopic external oblique anterior release as well as posterior release techniques such as the robotic transversus abdominis release (TAR). Finally, other useful variations of complex repair such as the robotic extended totally extraperitoneal (eTEP) approach will be described.

Keywords: abdominal wall reconstruction, component separation, hernia repair, robotic surgery, minimally invasive surgery

1. Introduction

The history of component separation starts at the beginning of the twentieth century, after the advent of general anesthesia in 1846. Thanks to the combined efforts and lessons learned from Charles Gibson, C.F. Dixon, and Donald Young, eventually Oscar Ramirez was able to describe his technique of abdominal fascial release and popularize the modern "component separation" technique.

Early efforts at primary closure of incisional hernias were prone to failure because of poor suture materials, inadequate prostheses, and most importantly, the tension on the repair. It was at the beginning of the twentieth century that Gibson described a method for "plastic repair of the abdominal wall" that involved relaxing incisions on the lateral anterior rectus sheath.

In 1929, Dixon modified Gibson's method and instead released the anterior rectus sheath 0.5 cm from its medial border bilaterally, turning over and opposing these fascial flaps in the midline [1–3].

In 1961, a more complex version of these techniques was described by Young when attempting closure of epigastric hernias, a common complication in the pre-laparoscopic era secondary to large incisions for open cholecystectomies and wound infections. Based on previous descriptions by Gibson and Dixon, Young advised separating the anterior and posterior rectus sheath from the rectus muscle to release the muscle and allow it to move easily to the midline. Next, the lateral border of the rectus sheath was incised a finger's breadth medial to the costal margin in the upper epigastrium and the same distance from the lateral edge of the rectus muscle in the lower epigastrium to reduce tension on the repair.

Ramirez, in his landmark article, described the component separation technique by releasing the external oblique aponeurosis lateral to the lateral edge of the rectus sheath. This is the critical maneuver of releasing the external oblique aponeurosis from the anterior rectus sheath lateral to the semilunar line. In 1990, Ramirez described what is now known as the modern component separation technique. After studying the technique in 10 fresh cadavers and applying the anatomic findings to reconstruct the abdominal wall defect of 11 patients, Ramirez published his technique in the journal of Plastic and Reconstructive Surgery. He described releasing the external oblique muscle through a lateral incision to the semilunar line and separating the external oblique muscle from the internal oblique muscle in a relatively avascular plane.

With the goal of restoring the normal anatomy of the abdominal wall at the midline, Ramirez incised the aponeurosis of the external oblique muscle lateral to the lateral edge of the rectus sheath and performed extensive dissection underneath the external oblique, separating it from the internal oblique muscle. Additionally, the rectus muscle was separated from the posterior rectus sheath at the midline. These dissections allowed the advancement of the "components" of the abdominal wall – the rectus abdominis, the external oblique, the internal oblique, and the transversus abdominis muscles – to the midline, allowing ventral hernia defects of 20 cm to be closed without tension [4].

2. Posterior release component separation

In the 1960s, Jean Rives and Rene Stoppa also developed the Rives Stoppa technique for retrorectus mesh repair known as the Rives-Stoppa method. In this repair, extensive dissection is carried out in the space between the rectus abdominis muscle and the posterior rectus sheath to create a space to place the mesh. This allows the rectus abdominis muscle to mobilize more toward the midline, but because the repair is limited by the lateral border of the posterior rectus sheath, it may be inadequate to repair larger hernias [5].

Outside of Ramirez's original description of the component separation, an additional approach to hernia repair was described later by Novitsky in 2012 known as the transversus abdominis release (TAR). This approach is an extension of the Rives-Stoppa technique and has quite a few advantages. The key component of this repair is to release the transversus abdominis muscle itself. There are several advantages to this approach. Release of the transversus abdominis allows medial mobilization of the posterior rectus sheath. The function of the transversus abdominis and posterior fibers of the internal oblique is to provide tension throughout the thoracolumbar fascia and increase abdominal fascia integrity. Therefore, since the muscles are almost circumferential, the dissection allows access to almost unlimited space, as described below. Novitsky described this in detail in his 2012 description [6–8].

After entering the abdomen via laparotomy, the posterior rectus sheath is identified and incised 0.5 to 1 cm medial to the anterior/posterior sheath junction to expose the transversus abdominis. Starting at the level of the umbilicus, the retromuscular place is developed laterally toward the linea semilunaris. During this dissection, the neurovascular bundles penetrating the lateral edge of the posterior rectus sheath can be visualized and must be preserved. The posterior rectus sheath is divided 0.5–1 cm medial from its edge. The retromuscular plan is developed toward the linea semilunaris and then incised in the upper abdomen to visualize the underlying transversus abdominis. The neurovascular bundles that are penetrating the posterior sheath are preserved. The entire length of the transversus abdominis is then incised with electrosurgical energy at its medial edge. This allows entrance to the space above the transversalis fascia. This plane can be dissected to reach the space of Retzius anterior to the urinary bladder, and the subxiphoid space superiorly. The large retrorectus space is closed by closing the posterior sheath with a running monofilament suture, after which a mesh is placed and secured. Of note, in Novitsky's experience, this technique allowed 8–12 cm of advancement per side toward the midline. This technique opened an entirely new plane to repair large abdominal hernias and is really a natural progression of the repairs described before this.

3. Minimally invasive TAPP and TEP

When the laparoscopic approach to ventral hernias was first introduced, the techniques described the placement of intraperitoneal underlay mesh later on called intraperitoneal onlay mesh (IPOM). Its implementation has been complicated by adhesive bowel disease, mesh erosion, and enterocutaneous fistulae from direct contact between the mesh and bowel. Due to these complications, a transabdominal preperitoneal (TAPP) approach was described. This technique involved entering the abdominal cavity laparoscopically and developing a preperitoneal/retrorectus space for placement of the mesh.

In 2018, Belyansky described a novel approach for approaching ventral hernia repair using a totally extraperitoneal technique, which previously had been described for laparoscopic inguinal hernia repairs. He called it the enhanced-view totally extraperitoneal (eTEP) technique which is also referred as the extended totally extraperitoneal technique. With this method of repair, laparoscopic ports are placed into the retrorectus space where dissection occurs first in one of the retrorectus spaces and then the contralateral one, which allows for placement of a retrorectus mesh similar to the Rives-Stoppa technique.

With the advent of robotic surgery and the dexterity provided by robotic instruments as compared to laparoscopic instruments, many surgeons have attempted repair of larger and more complex hernias.

4. Robotic reconstruction techniques

4.1 Robotic IPOM

The patient is placed in the supine position with both arms tucked and secured to avoid any movement during the procedure and to allow room for docking of the robot and avoidance of collision between the patient's arm and the robotic arm. Three ports are placed based on surgeon preference, but typically on the most lateral aspect of the abdominal wall, usually on the left side but not exclusively there. If the hernia is in the midline, these may be placed on either side. Our ports are placed at least 8 cm apart to avoid interference between the arms of the robotic instruments.

After port site selection, we typically gain entry into the abdomen using a 5 mm optical trocar and 0° laparoscope via the optical entry technique. Once pneumoperitoneum is obtained, the other two 8 mm robotic trocars are then placed under direct visualization. The original 5 mm port is substituted by an 8 mm robotic trocar which may be upsized to 12 mm if necessary during the case to introduce the mesh intraperitoneally according to the selected size. A 5 mm accessory port may also be placed to help assist the operative surgeon but is often unnecessary. With large hernia defects or when extensive lysis of adhesions is indicated, an assistant port or the fourth robotic arm may be helpful to aid in tissue retraction and facilitate a safe and timely dissection. The robot is then docked, and robotic instruments are introduced under direct visualization.

The first step in the procedure is adhesiolysis, if indicated. The difficulty varies from case to case depending on hernia size, chronicity, and prior procedures. Adhesions are taken down using a combination of blunt and sharp dissection. Electrosurgical energy may also be used at the surgeon's discretion, but care must be taken to avoid thermal injury to any vital structures contained in the hernia sac such as the intestine. The hernia contents are reduced back intraperitoneally, and inspection of the contents is done to confirm no damage has been done to any of the contents and further hemostasis is achieved. The fascial defect is then measured. Insufflation is reduced before measuring the defect to prevent overestimation of the hernia defect.

If feasible, the fascial defect is closed primarily. In our practice, we typically perform this in a continuous fashion using a permanent barbed suture. First, we bring down the insufflation from 15 to 8 mm Hg to reduce any tension on the primary closure. A non-absorbable barbed suture is introduced intraperitoneally. The fascia is then closed in a continuous fashion, although this could be done in an interrupted fashion per surgeon preference.

The next step is the placement of the mesh. Per the current literature, a 4–5 cm mesh overlap is recommended for ventral hernia repairs. After appropriate mesh selection, the mesh is rolled up extracorporeally and then introduced into the cavity using a 12 mm port. The mesh is then oriented so that it can overlap 4–5 cm circumferentially around the defect. The overlap is important due to future contraction of the mesh that occurs during the healing phase, which can lead to re-emergence of the defect and increased risk of hernia recurrence.

Once the mesh is in the appropriate position, fixation can be achieved by multiple methods as in laparoscopic surgery. These include intracorporeal suturing and tacking with different products. An advantage of the IPOM repair from a robotic approach is that the mesh can easily and reliably be fixated utilizing intracorporeal suturing due to the improved visualization, ergonomics, and dexterity that is achievable in robotic surgery. In our practice, the mesh is sutured using a non-absorbable monofilament barbed suture in a continuous, running fashion. Multiple sutures may need to be used depending on the size of the mesh. This is based on surgeon preference, but it may also be fixated in an interrupted fashion.

After the mesh has been placed, the abdomen is once again inspected to ensure hemostasis. The robotic instruments are removed under direct visualization and the robot is undocked. The 12 mm port is removed first, and the abdomen is desufflated to 8 mm Hg to reduce tension on the fascia. The fascial defect is closed primarily in a simple interrupted fashion using 0-Vicryl suture on a suture passer. The gas is turned off and the abdomen is desufflated followed by removal of the remaining ports. The skin is then closed using 4-0 Monocryl in a subcuticular fashion and Dermabond is applied over the skin closure sites [9–14].

4.2 Robotic IPOM with endoscopic anterior component separation

Another described technique for hernia repair is the endoscopic anterior (external oblique) component separation with robotic hernia repair. This procedure involves a two-stage approach.

In the first stage, an anterior component separation is performed on the external oblique aponeurosis endoscopically with laparoscopic instruments. Ports are placed lateral to the semilunar line. The space between the external and internal oblique aponeuroses is entered using a cut-down approach with sharp and blunt dissection. An intramural plane is initially dissected between these structures using a finger followed by a balloon spacer. Laparoscopic trocars are placed bilaterally. The laparoscope and monopolar scissors are then used to visualize and further dissect this plane to perform an open anterior component separation on the external oblique aponeurosis lateral to the semilunar line.

The second stage of the operation involves entering the peritoneal cavity via the optical trocar technique to carry out a robotic reduction and closure of the hernia defect as described above in the IPOM technique section. By performing endoscopic component separation before IPOM, primary repair of the defect before mesh placement is easier as these fascial planes have been released [15–17].

4.3 Robotic eTEP

The robotic retrorectus flap creation achieved with an extended totally extraperitoneal (eTEP) approach offers multiple advantages including the development of a tension-free repair, the lack of contact between the mesh and the underlying intraperitoneal viscera, and the position of the mesh in the preperitoneal plane, which eliminates the risk of future adhesion formation. The patient is placed in a supine position. Arms are tucked loosely to allow them to drift slightly posterior. This allows for an additional range of motion for the robotic arm to prevent the patient's arm from colliding with it. This also ensures that the superior-most port does not collide with the patient's arm when placed out laterally. Care is taken not to hyperextend the shoulder during positioning. Due to this positioning, one can also perform transversus abdominis release if necessary, from either side of the patient without having to reposition them.

Optical entry is performed in the left upper quadrant medial to the semilunar line by using a 5 mm optical entry port with care not to penetrate the posterior rectus sheath to avoid entering the peritoneal cavity (**Figure 1**). The posterior rectus sheath is visualized, and blunt dissection is carried out to develop this plane for subsequent insufflation. Pneumopreperitoneum is established to continue to develop the left retrorectus space ideally with an Airseal insufflation system to prevent loss of insufflation if a small defect is created accidentally on the posterior rectus sheath (**Figure 2**). A small amount of blunt dissection is carried out to enable placement of a second 5 mm port (Airseal) inferior to the initial port.

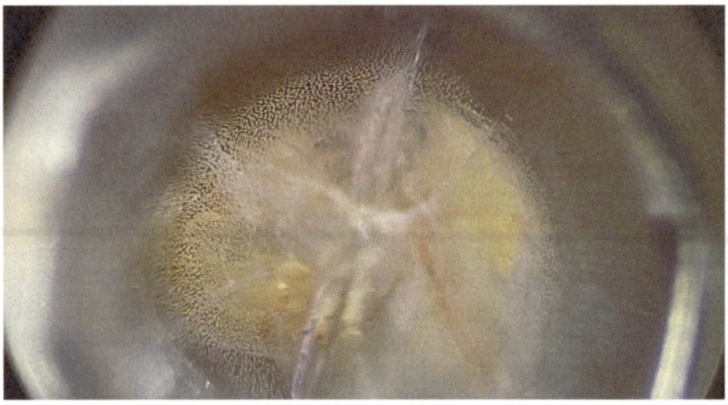

Figure 1.
Optical entry into the left retrorectus space.

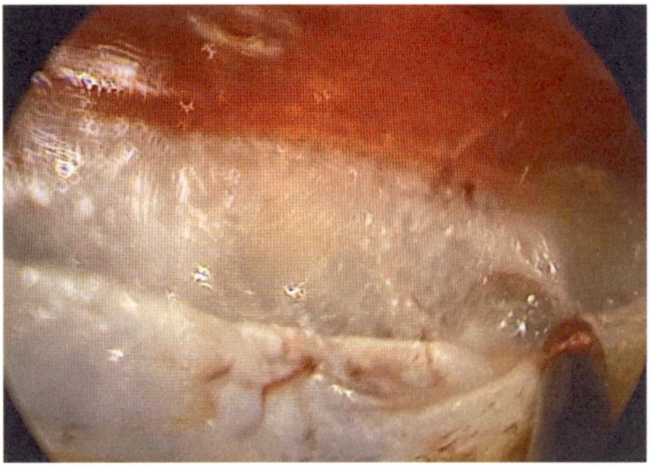

Figure 2.
Endoscopic development of left retrorectus flap.

Endoscopic dissection of areolar tissue with laparoscopic instruments including the monopolar electrosurgical hook is carried out superiorly/inferiorly and across the midline in the epigastric region by dividing the medial aspect of the left retrorectus space and crossing over to the right retrorectus space over the linea alba (**Figure 3**). During this step, rectus diastasis becomes obvious with this crossing-over maneuver to the right retrorectus space. This step is necessary to insert three 8 mm robotic trocars in a horizontal line disposition across the upper abdomen (**Figure 4**). One of these trocars can be upsized later to 12 mm to introduce the mesh. On the other hand, robotic trocars may be placed either superiorly or laterally depending on the desired approach and location of the hernia defect. If one is planning on performing an extensive transversus abdominis release (TAR) in addition to hernia repair via the eTEP approach, we recommend a superior port placement so that the bilateral TAR can be performed from the same port position without having to re-dock.

Continued dissection is carried out using monopolar electrosurgical energy with the robot to form a retromuscular plane of dissection around the hernia sac. One

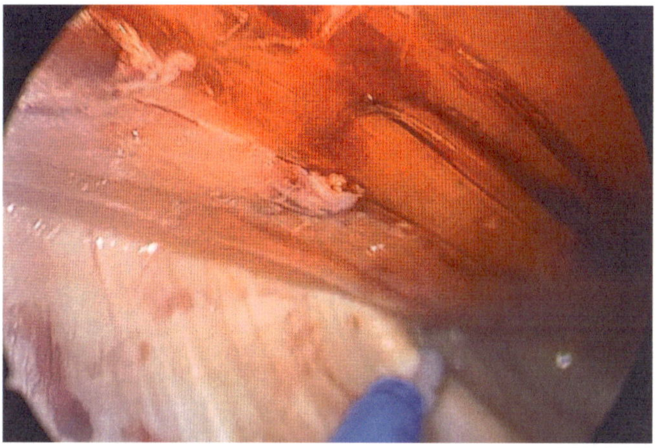

Figure 3.
Division of medial aspect of anterior rectus sheath to access the linea alba and cross the midline to the right anterior rectus sheath.

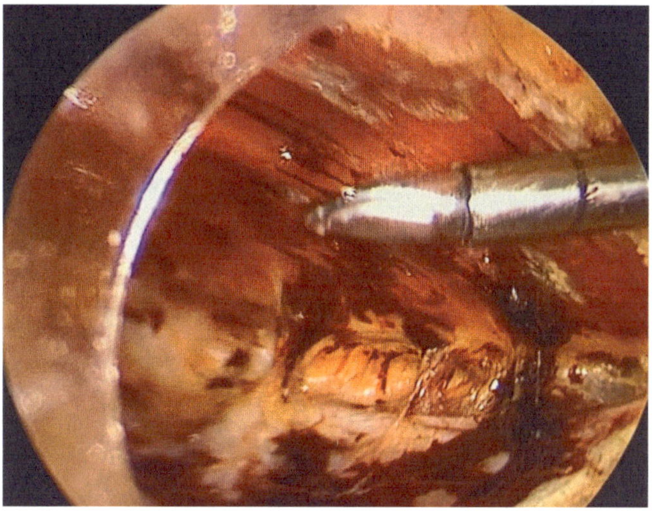

Figure 4.
Robotic trocar placement.

should be careful to avoid injuring neurovascular bundles penetrating the retromuscular plane. The lateral border of dissection is the semilunar line if not performing a concurrent TAR procedure.

The hernia sac is then reduced and, if necessary, opened carefully (**Figure 5**). One should avoid using electrosurgical energy during this portion of the procedure to avoid thermal injury to possible underlying bowel or other intraperitoneal structures. After reduction of contents, closure of the parietal peritoneum and the posterior sheath is performed with running barbed monofilament suture (**Figure 6**). The anterior aspect of the hernia fascial defect is then closed primarily and, if appropriate, the patient's rectus diastasis may be plicated at this time using the same suture used to close the hernia defect or a separate one. This is

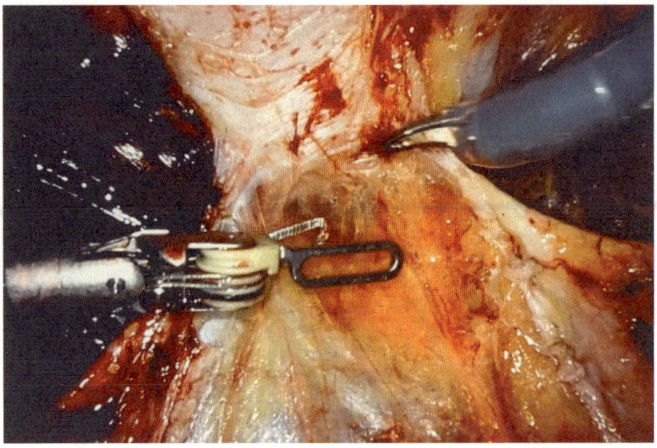

Figure 5.
Reduction of the hernia sac and contents.

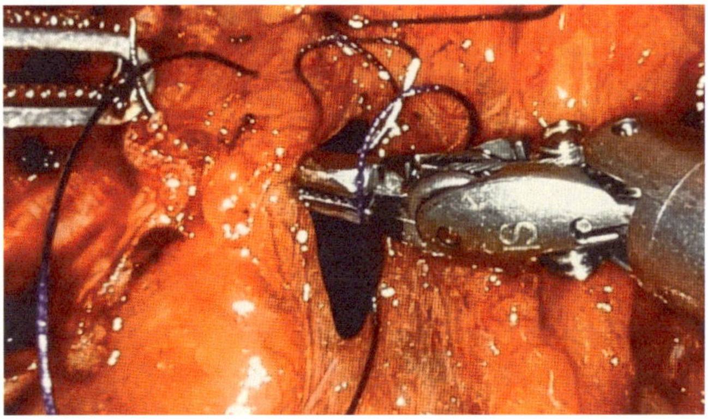

Figure 6.
Primary closure of peritoneal defects and posterior sheath.

an excellent opportunity to relieve the deformity caused by rectus diastasis and provide a plication and restoration of function to the abdominal wall with the hernia repair (**Figure** 7).

The cavity which has been dissected is measured to size the mesh appropriately. This may be accomplished by inserting a flexible ruler through a port and later retrieving it after measurement, or one can estimate the length using the 2.5 cm-long fenestrated bipolar grasper tip. Meticulous hemostasis is ensured before the insertion of mesh. If needed, hemostatic agents may be instilled into the cavity at this time. At our center, we prefer to use uncoated, nonabsorbable in this space if the procedure is performed in class 1 surgical wound, or uncoated biosynthetic hybrid mesh if the wound is class 2 or above with multiple risk factors such as obesity, type 2 diabetes, connective tissue disease, or advanced age with cardiovascular disease. The risk of contamination is minimized as the peritoneal space is not significantly violated except when reducing the hernia contents and the mesh is separated from the bowel by the transversalis and extraperitoneal fascia. Due to the

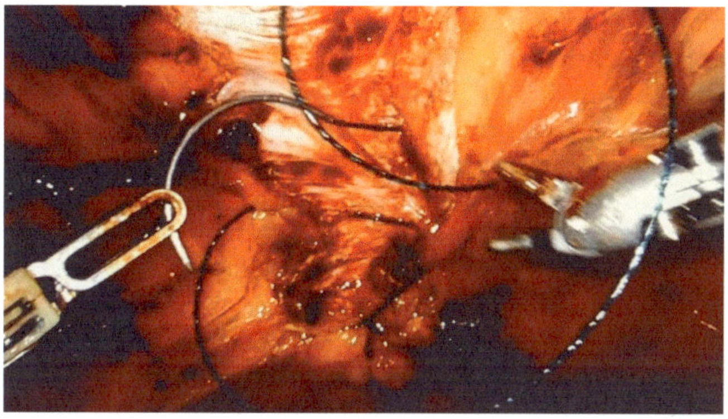

Figure 7.
Anterior fascial defect closure +/− rectus diastasis plication.

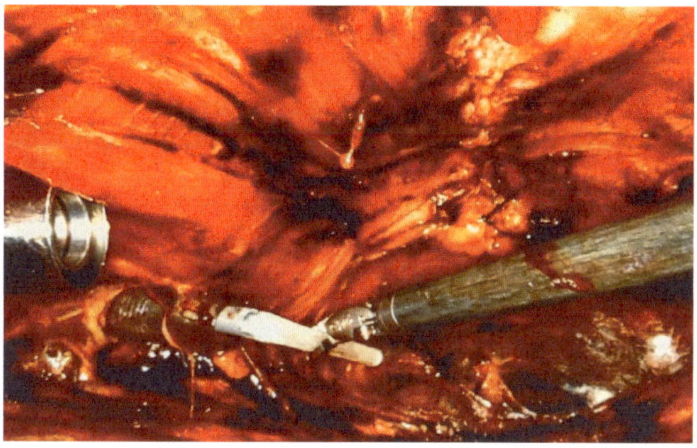

Figure 8.
Mesh introduction and deployment +/− hemostatic agent.

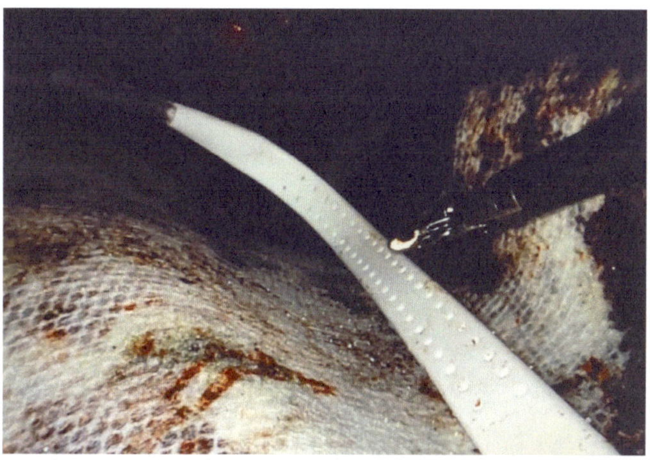

Figure 9.
Drain placement.

presence of fascial layers deep in the retromuscular space, coating of the mesh is not necessary as it does not contact the bowel.

After selection, the mesh is rolled up and inserted through one of the trocars using an atraumatic grasper **(Figure 8)**. If the mesh is too large to be inserted through an 8 mm port, one of the ports may need to be upsized to a 12 mm port. The use of a hemostatic agent or powder is helpful to prevent seroma and hematoma formation.

Since concern for hematoma or seroma formation exists, a closed suction surgical drain is placed in the retromuscular space prior to desufflation and removal of trocars **(Figure 9)**. The drain typically only stays for a week or two, since keeping it for a longer period of time may also be a nidus for infection. Finally, the retromuscular space is desufflated under direct vision and incisions are closed using Monocryl suture in a subcuticular fashion.

5. Robotic transversus abdominis release (TAR)

Similar to eTEP, the TAR technique offers a retrorectus dissection, but from a transabdominal/intraperitoneal approach and with the additional advantage of extending itself lateral to the semilunar line to release the muscle and facilitate a posterior component separation. The patient is placed in a supine position. Arms are tucked loosely to allow them to drift slightly posteriorly. This allows for an additional range of motion for the robotic arm to prevent the patient's arm from colliding with it. This also ensures that the superior-most port does not collide with the patient's arm when placed out laterally. Care is taken not to hyperextend the shoulder during positioning. Due to this positioning, one can also perform a transversus abdominis release from either side of the patient without having to reposition them.

Optical entry in the left upper quadrant utilizing a 5 mm laparoscopic port. Once pneumoperitoneum is obtained, an 8 mm robotic trocar is placed in the left lower abdomen and another in the left lateral abdomen. The original 5 mm laparoscopic

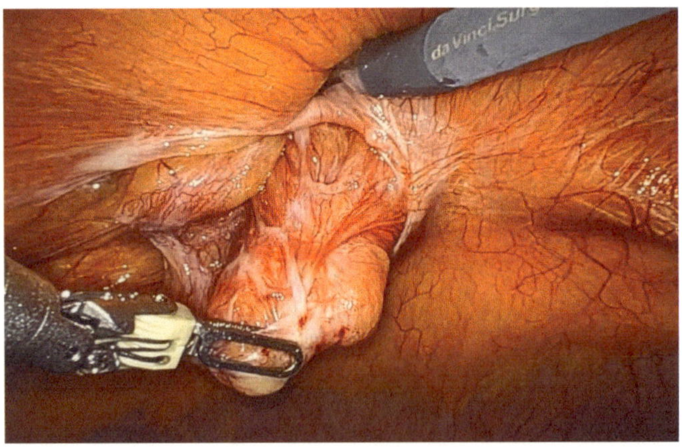

Figure 10.
Reduction of hernia sac and contents with adhesiolysis.

port is upsized for a 12 mm robotic trocar. The typical approach per our preference is from the left side of the abdominal wall to first develop the right retrorectus space from a transabdominal/intraperitoneal approach.

After general surveillance of the abdomen and robotic adhesiolysis if indicated, the hernia sac is reduced and the contralateral posterior rectus sheath is clearly identified (**Figure 10**). Depending on the size and extent of the falciform ligament, it may have to be mobilized superiorly (**Figure 11**).

Once the contralateral (right) posterior rectus sheath is clearly defined along the edge of the hernia defect, it is divided 0.5–1 cm medial from its edge to enter the plane where retrorectus dissection will take place. The contralateral retromuscular plane is developed laterally toward the linea semilunaris to the medial aspect of the lateral edge of the rectus abdominis, where the posterior sheath is divided in the upper abdomen just inferior to the ribcage to enter the proper plane and visualize the underlying transversus abdominis (**Figure 12**). The neurovascular

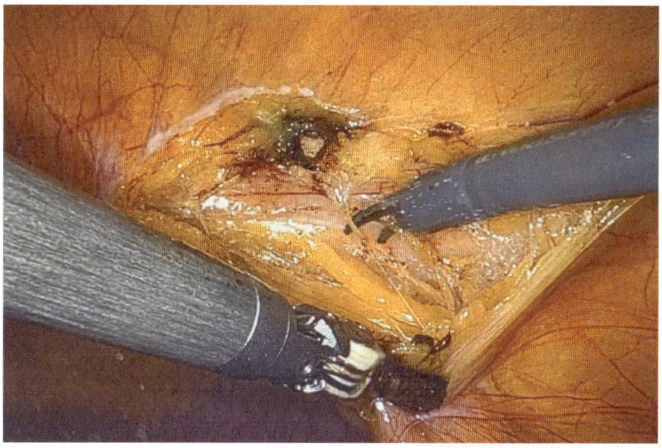

Figure 11.
Superior mobilization of falciform ligament.

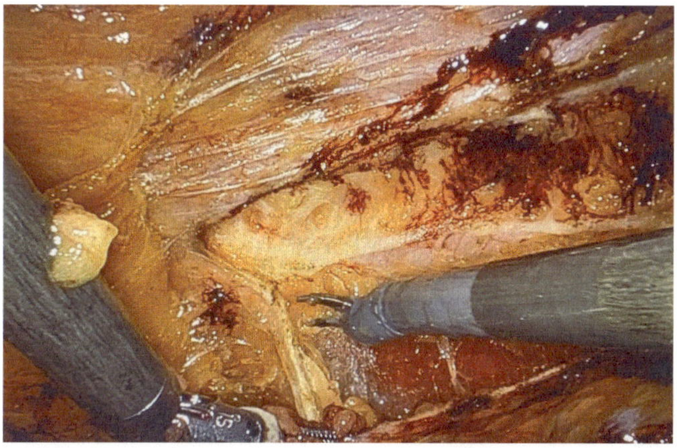

Figure 12.
Right retrorectus flap creation with preservation of neurovascular bundles.

bundles that are penetrating the posterior sheath are preserved. The entire length of the transversus abdominis is then incised with electrosurgical energy at its medial edge. This allows entrance to the space above the transversalis fascia and is carried out 2 cm lateral to the linea semilunaris. This plane can be dissected to reach the space of Retzius anteriorly to the urinary bladder, and the subxiphoid space superiorly **(Figure 13)**.

Once a satisfactory retrorectus space is developed, mirror image steps are repeated on the opposite site **(Figure 14)** including the position of the ports **(Figure 15)**. There will be a total of three 8 mm robotic trocars placed on the right side of the abdomen.

The floor of the large retrorectus space is reconstructed after the bilateral TAR posterior component separation by closing the posterior sheath with a running barbed monofilament suture in a running fashion **(Figure 16)**. This step can be performed tension-free due to the component separation bilaterally.

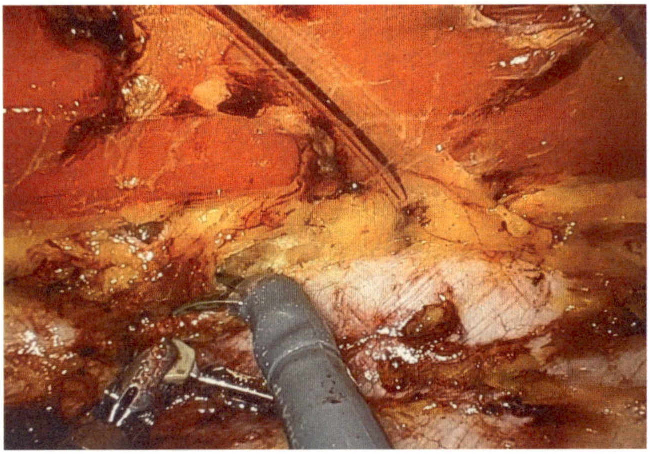

Figure 13.
Right TAR at 2 cm lateral to semilunar line.

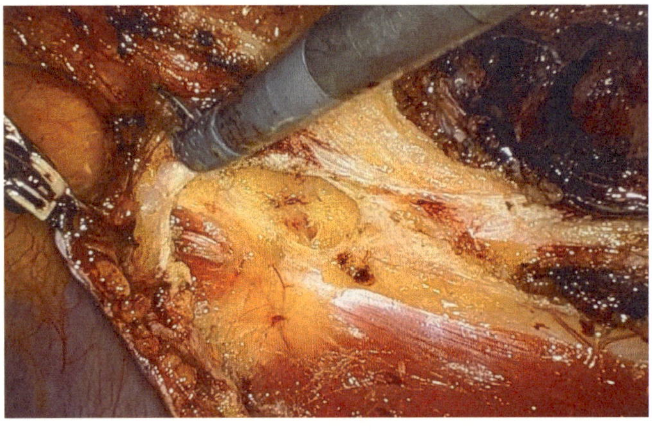

Figure 14.
Left retrorectus flap creation with preservation of neurovascular bundles.

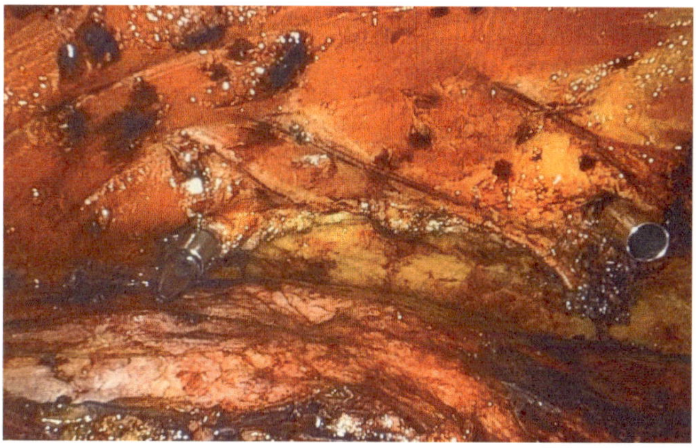

Figure 15.
Right abdominal wall port insertion before flipping the boom.

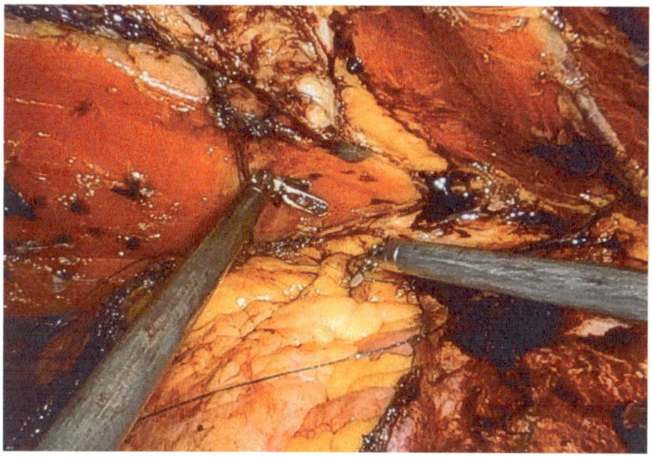

Figure 16.
Posterior sheath/peritoneum closure.

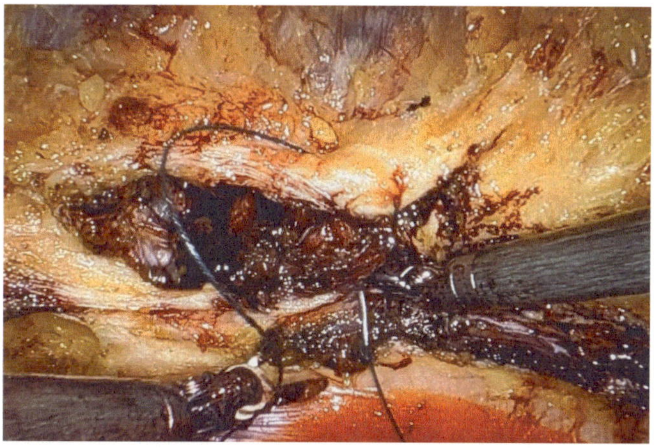

Figure 17.
Anterior fascial closure +/− rectus diastasis plication.

The next portion involves closure of the anterior fascial defect corresponding with the hernia and rectus diastasis plication (if present) with a running barbed monofilament suture **(Figure 17)**.

A preperitoneal mesh is introduced via a 12 mm robotic port in the left upper quadrant **(Figure 18)** and it is deployed over the now-closed posterior rectus sheath **(Figure 19)**. Above the mesh is the closed anterior fascial repair. There is no need to suture the mesh because it will remain in place between the muscle layers and fascial layers.

Hemostatic agent powder is placed over the mesh to promote adhesion of the mesh and reduce the incidence of seroma/hematoma. A total of two surgical drains are placed over the mesh to capture the extra fluid that would be produced in the newly formed space and prevent a seroma formation **(Figure 20)**. The drains exit via the upper quadrant incisions and are secured to the skin with a suture.

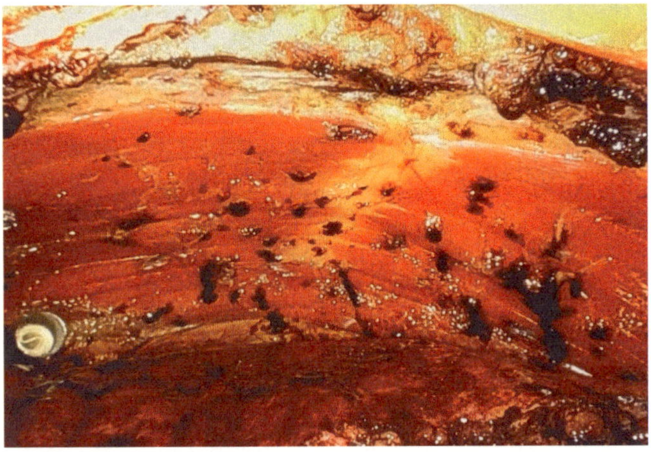

Figure 18.
Mesh introduction +/− hemostatic agent.

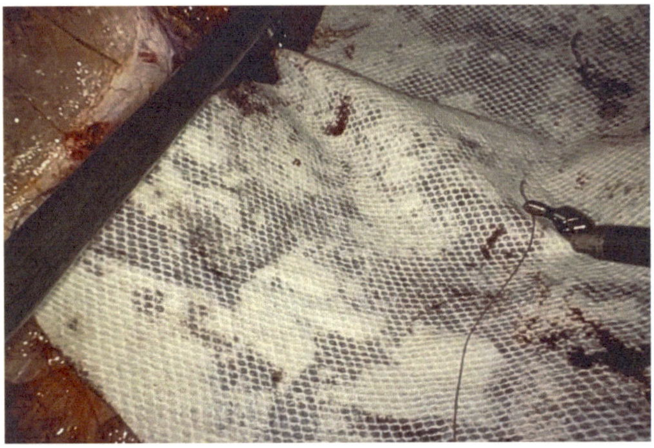

Figure 19.
Mesh positioning in preperitoneal space.

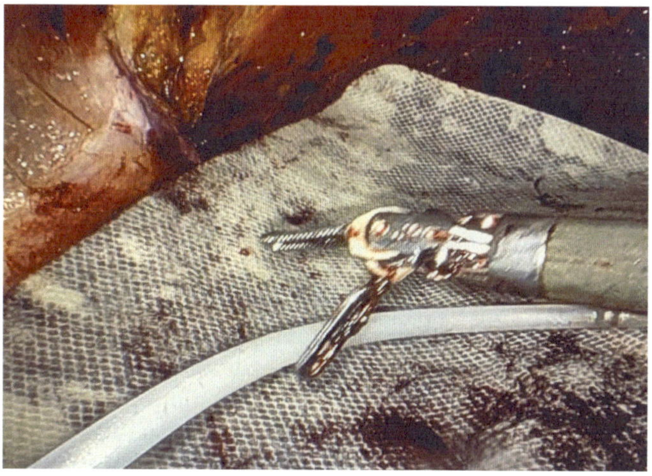

Figure 20.
Bilateral drain insertion.

6. Complications and management

Robotic ventral hernia repair is considered a safe and durable procedure. Indeed, open, endoscopic/laparoscopic, and robotic-assisted approaches are effective for ventral hernia repair with comparable overall outcomes. Nevertheless, each approach may demonstrate different advantages and disadvantages. Published data demonstrate that patients undergoing robotic ventral hernia repair have a significantly shorter hospital length of stay, lower conversion rate, and a lower rate of complications compared to the laparoscopic approach. Moreover, the robotic approach has a lower 30-day reoperation rate and a similar operative time in comparison to the open approach. On the other hand, the laparoscope approach has a shorter operative time and is less expensive than the robotic technique [18–21].

The abdominal wall reconstruction, like any surgical procedure, can be prone to complications. These could be related directly to the procedure, or they may be nonspecific regardless of the type of surgery. Pre-operative risk assessment and post-operative strategies could lead to a reduction in the complication rate and must be considered in every patient. In this context, the development of the robotic approach is due to its performance in high-risk cases. It is well suited for patients with risk factors such as morbid obesity and diabetes where microvascular disease and effects on the blood supply interfere with the healing of the abdominal wall. Moreover, patients with previous hernia repair by open surgery, connective tissue diseases, and rectus diastasis can take advantage of this new technique.

Despite the benefits and efficiency of the minimally invasive technique and the component separation procedure, several complications can pose postoperative challenges for the patient and surgical team [22–29]. Seroma and hematoma represent two of the most common postoperative complications after ventral hernia repair. However, since they have been described in the literature following different parameters, their real clinical incidence is variable. Seroma consists of an accumulation of clear fluid under the skin and usually develops where larger parts of tissue have been removed. It often has a minimal impact on the patient, but sometimes it could result in patient dissatisfaction, discomfort, poor esthetic outcome, and surgical site infections.

Moreover, major seroma-related complications could lead to deep infection, mesh rejection, and hernia recurrence. Asymptomatic seroma can be managed conservatively, but esthetic complaints, complications, symptomatic, and chronic forms require medical treatment. The first-line treatment should be the drainage of the liquid, eventually followed by repeated aspirations and a microbiological examination if an infectious process is suspected. If this approach is not effective, it might need an operative intervention with drainage of the fluid and removal of the pseudo-capsule.

Among the most common complications, there are surgical site infections (SSIs), including superficial, deep, or mesh infections. Independent predictors of SSI could be steroid use, prolonged operative time, and smoking. SSI can represent a dangerous postoperative complication and is a significant risk factor for recurrence. Furthermore, soft tissue infection is a serious, life-threatening condition that could lead to necrosis of the skin, muscles, and soft tissues. Most superficial infections can be treated with antibiotics plus accurate and regular wound care. Chronic superficial and deep mesh infections require a surgical approach because antibiotics alone typically have a poor success rate considering the bacteria's biofilm around the mesh that protects them. Debridement and lavage of the wound delineate the first crucial step followed by explanation of the infected mesh material, even if this maneuver causes secondary trauma to the abdominal wall and might be associated with a higher risk of complications. Microbiological analysis of the fluid surrounding the mesh is necessary for post-operative specific antibiotic therapy.

Besides the infectious process, the mesh can trigger a non-infectious reaction characterized by inflammation, fibrosis, and calcification. This phenomenon called "foreign body reaction" consists of an autoimmune response to a foreign body, producing organized granulation tissue. Specifically, the pathophysiology is explained by the attraction and stimulation of macrophages, which release cytokines, growth factors, matrix-modulating factors, and complement activating factors. Depending on the mesh used, the chronic granulomas could be more extensive and create a thick collagenous scar adherent to the abdominal wall. Indeed, they are characterized by an increased cell turnover that continues for periods of several years after the implantation of the mesh. Usually, the clinical manifestations could be a rejection or migration of the mesh, characterized by chronic pain [30, 31].

During an abdominal wall reconstruction, some tissues may be injured. Especially superficial and deep nerve structures and muscle components are at greater risk. If cutaneous nerves are damaged during the incision, these can take a notably long time to heal, and they may never completely recover. This situation implies a total or partial loss of sensation in localized areas. Moreover, even if muscle atrophy is often a direct consequence of incisions, sutures, or reduced blood supply, it is also associated with denervation. For all these reasons, abdominal surgery could be linked to a dysfunctional abdominal wall musculature. While denervation is more difficult to treat, transected muscles such as external and internal oblique or transversus abdominis could be reconstructed primarily and repaired with mesh.

Intestinal disorders are part of the possible complications of complex abdominal wall reconstruction. Defective hernia mesh positioning, post-operative scar tissue, or adhesions can cause a mechanical blockage that generates bowel obstructions. These are clinically highlighted as colicky pain, constipation, nausea, and vomiting. Furthermore, as in all abdominal surgeries, there is a risk that the abdomen temporarily loses its usual rhythmic contraction. The loss of peristaltic capacity, defined as paralytic ileus, is, in any case, a temporary condition and lasts from a few hours to a few days. Rarely, bowel injury can also happen, but this is most often due to a direct injury during port insertion or handling of the bowel with instruments such as during adhesiolysis.

Chronic pain and hernia recurrence are the most common long-term complications. Chronic pain remains difficult to evaluate and is usually defined as pain persisting for more than 3 months after surgery. More precisely, its clinical manifestations are mainly represented as increased sensitivity to pain and pain secondary to normally non-painful tactile stimuli. Some risk factors are preoperative pain, female sex, smoke, and younger age. The pathophysiology of neuropathic pain is explained sometimes by a surgical injury to a major nerve or an inflammation of the nerve as an adverse effect of mesh implantation. The injured and inflammatory cells release cytokines, bradykinin, and prostaglandins that activate nociceptors. Chronic pain is considered one of the most important factors for satisfaction, and its management depends on the proper identification of the etiology. Moreover, the experience of pain is more than the detection of noxious stimuli, social environment, and psychosocial factors should be considered alongside in the management of the patient. Concerning neuropathic cutaneous pain, medical treatment as topical lidocaine or capsaicin can help to block the conduction of impulses along nerves, by minimizing the transmission of pain. Oral drugs such as anticonvulsants, tricyclic antidepressants, serotonin-norepinephrine reuptake inhibitors can be used, too [32–34].

Morbidly obese and diabetic patients, those suffering from cardiovascular disease, immunosuppressed patients due to a prior transplant or immunocompromised for other reasons, and patients who underwent a prior hernia repair in a contaminated environment have a high risk of recurrence. All of the typical post-operative complications such as wound infection, seroma, hematoma, and wound dehiscence are present in these groups with several risk factors. A minimally invasive approach, including robotics, becomes relevant and crucial to the success of abdominal wall reconstruction in these patients.

To treat the recurrence of a hernia, choosing the optimal surgical treatment is of paramount importance. The surgeon must take into consideration various factors such as the technique previously used, the number of interventions and relapses, and other patient factors, such as smoking. Robotic ventral hernia repair has shown a low recurrence rate at a mean of 21 months postoperatively. Furthermore, it represents an optimal option for the treatment of complex recurrences considering the benefits of the minimally invasive surgical approach as well as increased dexterity and three-dimensional visualization. Indeed, this precision approach is often required for a correct and integral abdominal wall reconstruction, restoring the displaced tissues to normal anatomy and dynamics with a meticulous component separation to release the tension on the muscles and fascia. The rebuilding and restoration of a functional abdominal wall with the reinforcement offered by a robotic complex repair such as eTEP or TAR offers a durable, lifelong reconstruction to the patient [35, 36].

7. Conclusion

The techniques and approaches described in this chapter have evolved over time as a result of contributions from a collective group of surgeons who built their legacy upon the lessons learned from their predecessors. A robotic complex abdominal wall reconstruction is a highly demanding and technically specialized type of operation, but it does not mean that it should only be reserved for a certain category of surgeons. We strongly believe that all surgeons should be able to master these techniques with proper training, supervision, mentoring, and dedication to excellence and attention to detail. The relationship between anatomy and physiology becomes clear and obvious when a robotic abdominal wall reconstruction is performed to restore the mechanics and functionality that once existed in the human body before the development of a hernia. To learn how to achieve this monumental task takes a lifetime of perseverance and discipline, but it all starts with the desire to acquire this knowledge. This chapter intends to encourage its readers to enter the realm of robotic abdominal wall reconstruction with the highest purpose in mind: the highest possible quality of life that we can offer to our patients.

Author details

Rodolfo J. Oviedo[1,2,3,4*], Jeffrey Hodges[4], Joseph Nguyen-Lee[4], David Detz[4], Mary Oh[4], João Bombardelli[4], Anuj Shah[4], Atteeba Manzar[4] and Alessandro Martinino[5]

1 Houston Methodist Academic Institute, Houston, TX, United States

2 Texas A&M University College of Medicine, Bryan, TX, United States

3 Houston Methodist Research Institute, Houston, TX, United States

4 Houston Methodist Department of Surgery, Houston, TX, United States

5 Faculty of Medicine, Sapienza University of Rome, Rome, Italy

*Address all correspondence to: rjoviedo@houstonmethodist.org

IntechOpen

© 2022 The Author(s). Licensee IntechOpen. This chapter is distributed under the terms of the Creative Commons Attribution License (http://creativecommons.org/licenses/by/3.0), which permits unrestricted use, distribution, and reproduction in any medium, provided the original work is properly cited.

References

[1] Gibson CL. Post-operative Intestinal Obstruction. Annals of Surgery. 1916; **63**(4):442-451

[2] Dixon CF. Repair of incisional hernia. Surgery, Gynecology & Obstetrics. 1929;**48**:700-701

[3] Young D. Repair of Epigastric Incisional Hernia. The British Journal of Surgery. 1961;**48**:514-516

[4] Ramirez OM, Ruas E, Dellon AL. "Components Separation" method for closure of abdominal-wall defects: An anatomic and clinical study. Plastic and Reconstructive Surgery. 1990;**86**(3):519-526

[5] Stoppa RE. The treatment of complicated groin and incisional hernias. World Journal of Surgery. 1989;**13**:545-554

[6] Halvorson EG. On the origins of components separation. Plastic and Reconstructive Surgery. 2009; **124**(5):1545-1549

[7] Pereira X, Lima DL, Friedmann P, Romero-Velez G, Mandujano CC, Ramos-Santillan V, et al. Robotic abdominal wall repair: Adoption and early outcomes in a large academic medical center. Journal of Robotic Surgery. 2021;**20**:1-10

[8] Novitsky YW, Elliott HL, Orenstein SB, Rosen MJ. Transversus abdominis muscle release: A novel approach to posterior component separation during complex abdominal wall reconstruction. American Journal of Surgery. 2012;**204**(5):709-716

[9] Belyansky I, Daes J, Radu VG, Balasubramanian R, Reza Zahiri H, Weltz AS, et al. A novel approach using the enhanced-view totally extraperitoneal (eTEP) technique for laparoscopic retromuscular hernia repair. Surgical Endoscopy. 2018;**32**(3):1525-1532

[10] Barrera K, Chung P, Shraga S, Sugiyama G. Robotic ventral hernia repair. In: Derbel F, editor. Hernia. Rijeka: InTech; 2017

[11] Berger D. Laparoscopic IPOM technique. Der Chirurg; Zeitschrift Fur Alle Gebiete Der Operativen Medizen. 2010;**81**(3):211-215

[12] Bittner R, Bain K, Bansal VK, Berrevoet F, Bingener-Casey J, Chen D, et al. Update of Guidelines for laparoscopic treatment of ventral and incisional abdominal wall hernias. International Endohernia Society (IEHS)-Part A. Surgical Endoscopy. 2019;**33**(10):3069-3139

[13] Olmi S, Millo P, Piccoli M, Garulli G, Junior Nardi M, Pecchini F, et al. Laparoscopic treatment of incisional and ventral hernia. JSLS. 2021;**25**(2):e2021.00007

[14] Sauerland S, Walgenbach M, Habermalz B, Seiler CM, Miserez M. Laparoscopic versus open surgical techniques for ventral or incisional hernia repair. Cochrane Database of Systematic Reviews. 2011;**3**:CD007781

[15] Lowe JB, Garza JR, Bowman JL, Rohrich RJ, Strodel WE. Endoscopically assisted "components separation" for closure of abdominal wall defects. Plastic and Reconstructive Surgery. 2000;**105**(2):720-729

[16] Dauser B, Ghaffari S, Ng C, Schmid T, Köhler G, Herbst F.

Endoscopic anterior component separation: A novel technical approach. Hernia. Dec 2017;**21**(6):951-955

[17] Oviedo RJ, Robertson JC, Desai AS. Robotic ventral hernia repair and endoscopic component separation: Outcomes. JSLS. 2017;**21**(3):e2017.00055

[18] Coakley KM, Sims SM, Prasad T, Lincourt AE, Augenstein VA, Sing RF, et al. A nationwide evaluation of robotic ventral hernia surgery. American Journal of Surgery. 2017;**214**(6):1158-1163

[19] Altieri MS, Yang J, Xu J, Talamini M, Pryor A, Telem DA. Outcomes after robotic ventral hernia repair: A study of 21,565 patients in the state of New York. The American Surgeon. 2018;**84**(6):902-908

[20] Gonzalez A, Escobar E, Romero R, Walker G, Mejias J, Gallas M, et al. Robotic-assisted ventral hernia repair: A multicenter evaluation of clinical outcomes. Surgical Endoscopy. 2017;**31**(3):1342-1349

[21] LeBlanc KA, Gonzalez A, Dickens E, Olsofka J, Ortiz-Ortiz C, Verdeja J-C, et al. Robotic-assisted, laparoscopic, and open incisional hernia repair: Early outcomes from the prospective hernia study. Hernia. 2021;**25**(4):1071-1082

[22] Carbonell AM, Cobb WS, Chen SM. Posterior components separation during retromuscular hernia repair. Hernia. 2008;**12**(4):359-362

[23] Lopez-Monclus J, Muñoz-Rodríguez J, San Miguel C, Robin A, Blazquez LA, Pérez-Flecha M, et al. Combining anterior and posterior component separation for extreme cases of abdominal wall reconstruction. Hernia. 2020;**24**(2):369-379

[24] de Vries Reilingh TS, van Goor H, Rosman C, Bemelmans MH, de Jong D, van Nieuwenhoven EJ, et al. "Components separation technique" for the repair of large abdominal wall hernias. Journal of the American College of Surgeons. 2003;**196**(1):32-37

[25] Blair LJ, Cox TC, Huntington CR, Groene SA, Prasad T, Lincourt AE, et al. The effect of component separation technique on quality of life (QOL) and surgical outcomes in complex open ventral hernia repair (OVHR). Surgical Endoscopy. 2017;**31**(9):3539-3546

[26] Iqbal CW, Pham TH, Joseph A, Mai J, Thompson GB, Sarr MG. Long-term outcome of 254 complex incisional hernia repairs using the modified rives-stoppa technique. World Journal of Surgery. 2007;**31**(12):2398-2404

[27] Novitsky YW, Porter JR, Rucho ZC, Getz SB, Pratt BL, Kercher KW, et al. Open preperitoneal retrofascial mesh repair for multiply recurrent ventral incisional hernias. Journal of the American College of Surgeons. 2006;**203**(3):283-289

[28] Novitsky YW, Fayezizadeh M, Majumder A, Neupane R, Elliott HL, Orenstein SB. Outcomes of posterior component separation with transversus abdominis muscle release and synthetic mesh sublay reinforcement. Annals of Surgery. 2016;**264**(2):226-232

[29] Wegdam JA, Thoolen JMM, Nienhuijs SW, de Bouvy N, de Vries Reilingh TS. Systematic review of transversus abdominis release in complex abdominal wall reconstruction. Hernia. 2019;**23**(1):5-15

[30] Falagas ME, Kasiakou SK. Mesh-related infections after hernia repair surgery. Clinical Microbiology and Infection. 2005;**11**(1):3-8

[31] Heymann F, Trotha K-T v, Preisinger C, Lynen-Jansen P,

Roeth AA, Geiger M, et al. Polypropylene mesh implantation for hernia repair causes myeloid cell–driven persistent inflammation. JCI Insight. 2019;**4**(2):e123862. DOI: 10/1172/jci.insight.123862

[32] Cox TC, Huntington CR, Blair LJ, Prasad T, Lincourt AE, Heniford BT, et al. Predictive modeling for chronic pain after ventral hernia repair. American Journal of Surgery. 2016;**212**(3):501-510

[33] Tsirline VB, Colavita PD, Belyansky I, Zemlyak AY, Lincourt AE, Heniford BT. Preoperative pain is the strongest predictor of postoperative pain and diminished quality of life after ventral hernia repair. The American Surgeon. 2013;**79**(8):829-836

[34] Reddi D, Curran N. Chronic pain after surgery: Pathophysiology, risk factors and prevention. Postgraduate Medical Journal. 2014;**90**(1062):222-227

[35] Sharbaugh ME, Patel PB, Zaman JA, Ata A, Feustel P, Singh K, et al. Robotic ventral hernia repair: A safe and durable approach. Hernia. 2021;**25**(2):305-312

[36] Goettman MA, Riccardi ML, Vang L, Dughayli MS, Faraj CH. Robotic assistance in ventral hernia repair may decrease the incidence of hernia recurrence. Journal of Minimal Access Surgery. 2020;**16**(4):335-340

Chapter 11

Laparoscopic Hiatal Hernia Repair during in-Sleeve Gastrectomy

Seyfi Emir, Hasan Erdem, Mehmet Gençtürk, Muhammed Said Dalkılıç, Abdullah Şişik and Selim Sözen

Abstract

Obesity is one of the most important health problems in developed and developing countries. Morbid obesity is defined as having a body mass index (BMI) of more than 40 kg/m^2. Obesity does not only predispose to gastroesophageal reflux, but is also an important independent risk factor for the development of hiatal hernia (HH). There are articles advocating about half of obese patients have a hiatal hernia. Hiatal hernia not only exacerbates reflux symptoms, but may also lead to incomplete removal of the gastric fundus during laparoscopic sleeve gastrectomy (LSG). When hiatal hernias are seen preoperatively or intraoperatively for bariatric surgery, surgical correction should ideally be made with mesh reinforcement to prevent further clinical progression.

Keywords: obesity, laparoscopic sleeve gastrectomy, gastroesophageal reflux and hiatal hernia

1. Introduction

Obesity has an important place among the most important health problems of developed and developing countries [1–3]. If the body mass index (BMI), calculated by evaluating the height and weight together, is greater than 40 kg/m^2, it is called morbid obesity. Along with obesity, the risk of systemic diseases such as diabetes mellitus (DM), obstructive sleep apnea and cardiovascular diseases increases, resulting in an increase in mortality rates. However, one of the independent risk factors for the development of gastroesophageal reflux disease (GERD) is obesity. In addition to predisposing to gastroesophageal reflux, one of the important independent risk factors for the development of hiatal hernia (HH) is obesity [4–8].

On the other side, the hiatal hernia (HH) is closely related to the presence of GERD.

2. Discussion

Gastroesophageal reflux disease (GERD) and HH have a relatively high incidence in the morbidly obese population, the underlying pathophysiology is transient lower esophageal sphincter relaxation in combination with increased intra-abdominal pressure [9].

It has been proven that obesity is an important independent risk factor for the development of GERD and/or HH; while approximately 50–70% of patients undergoing bariatric surgery for morbid obesity have symptomatic reflux, 15% of them have symptomatic HH. GERD and HH are closely related with high BMI [10]. There are studies indicating the prevalence of GERD (defined as an increase in acid exposure and/or fissures in the esophageal mucosa) as 41% before laparoscopic sleeve gastrectomy (LSG) and 71% after LSG [11, 12].

There are articles advocating about half of obese patients have a hiatal hernia [5, 13]. Hiatal hernia not only exacerbates reflux symptoms, but may also lead to incomplete removal of the gastric fundus during LSG [3]. With the increasing use of LSG, more patients have been observed with relatively common side effects such as GERD and other somewhat rare anatomical complications such as strictures, ulcerations, and HH [14]. Small esophageal sliding herniation of LSG is thought to be associated with GERD after LSG, therefore surgical repair of HH is advocated by many [15]. Gastric narrowing, progressive enlargement of the esophageal hiatal opening, division of natural connections such as the phrenoesophageal membrane, and removal of the gastric fundus near the angle of His are possible factors associated with postoperative weight loss and reduction in visceral fat, and intrathoracic migration of the stomach [16]. Some authors have suggested that previous hiatal hernia repair (HHR) may accelerate postoperative LSG migration due to hiatal dissection, which may lead to phreno-esophageal membrane disruption, gastric sleeve instability, and associated loss of antireflux mechanisms [17].

In a study by Daes et al., it was found that hiatal hernia was detected intraoperatively in 25% of patients undergoing LSG, and reflux symptoms were significantly reduced after hiatal hernia repair (HHR) [18]. Baumann et al. [16], using multisection computed tomography, monitored 27 patients with gastric sleeve and they found that the migration of the staple line to the thorax is associated with the presence of gastroesophageal reflux. Interestingly, they demonstrated a 37% migration rate of the gastric sleeve into the posterior mediastinum 1–10 months after surgery. While 40% of these patients complained of reflux symptoms, 60% were asymptomatic. Most studies like this show an improvement in GERD when the hernia is repaired [19].

In the light of this information, if the presence of a hiatal hernia is known before bariatric surgery or if a hiatal hernia is detected during surgery, it is recommended to repair it [20–22]. In bariatric surgery, if it is detected in the preoperative evaluation or intraoperatively, concomitant repair should be performed [23, 24]. The repair of hiatal hernia during a gastric sleeve due to morbid obesity decreases the prevalence of GERD. It was revealed that dyspeptic symptoms and reflux symptoms regressed after HHR and that proton pump inhibitor usage declined. Unsuccessful hiatal hernia repair (HHR) can lead to an exacerbation of reflux symptoms after surgery. There are authors who advocate anterior and posterior placement of sutures in HHR to prevent anterior hiatal dilation during weight loss [25]. There are also articles in the literature reporting that HHR was performed safely with a mesh after LSG [26, 27].

3. Management and treatment

Fundoplication after bariatric surgery is not technically possible due to the lack of excess stomach tissue due to previous sleeve gastrectomy. Mesh reinforcement has been proven to have a lower incidence of recurrence than primary repair. Although there is no difference in complication rates between synthetic and biological mesh, it has been proven that synthetic mesh has a lower recurrence rate compared to biological mesh [28].

A randomized controlled trial conducted by Snyder at al [29] showed no difference between repairing and not performing HH during sleeve gastrectomy. Santonicola et al. [30] showed the results of repairing HH during gastric sleeve in 78 patients. The incidence of preoperative reflux was 38.4%, and 30.8% after 15 months of follow-up (p = 0.3). Dakour Aridi et al. studied the safety of repairing HH during gastrectomy [31]. The 28,000 patients who had only sleeve gastrectomy and 4687 patients who had sleeve gastrectomy + HH repair recorded in the database of the National Surgical Quality Improvement Program were compared. Examined groups were not different from each other in terms of complications and mortality. In fact, there were no

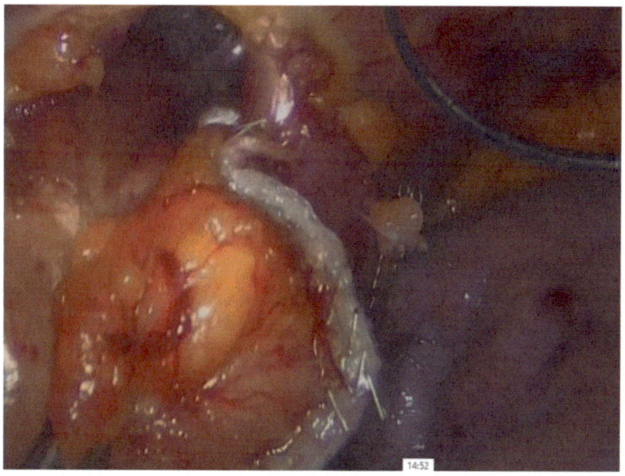

Figure 1.
Large hiatus/sleeve stapled line.

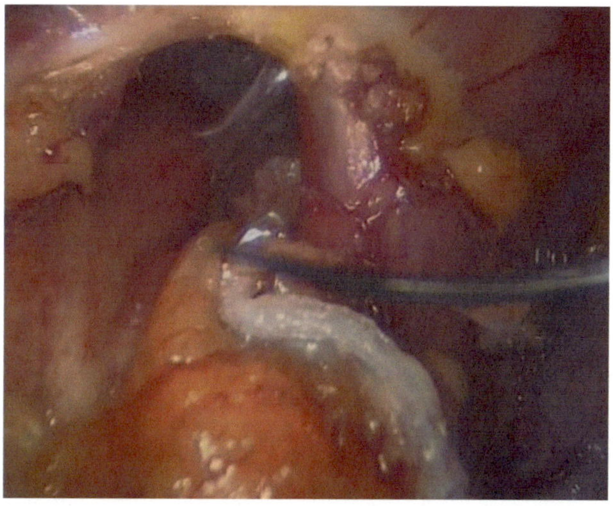

Figure 2.
Laparoscopic view of gastric sleeve herniation through esophageal hiatus.

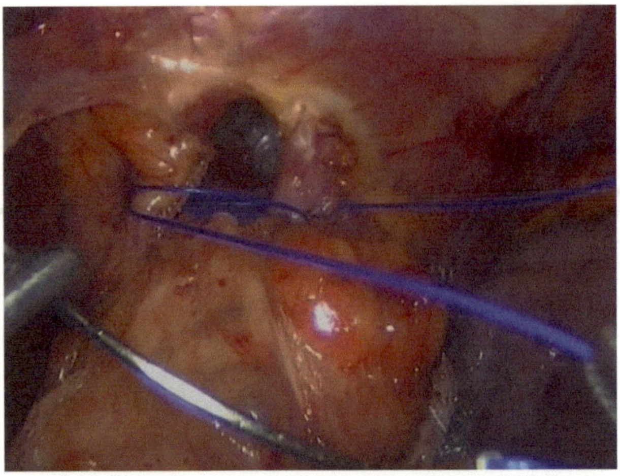

(a)

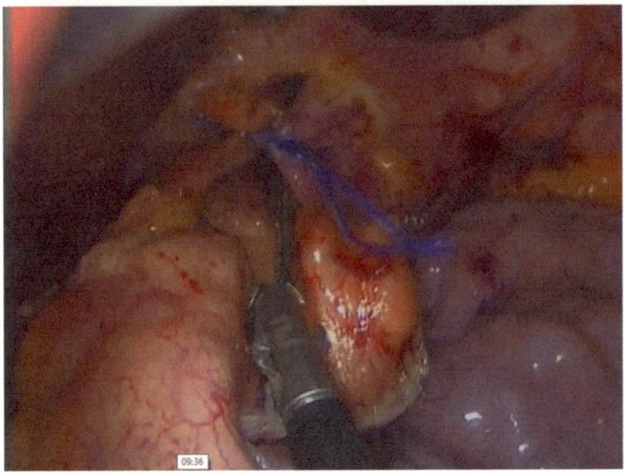

(b)

Figure 3.
(a) Laparoscopic view hiatal hernia repair. (b) Final aspect closed esophageal hiatus.

unexpected or adverse outcomes of performing esophageal dissection and performing hiatus repair. In addition, some anatomical and physiological results of sleeve gastrectomy surgery can explain the regression in preoperative symptoms. With LSG, the total gastric mucosal surface and, accordingly, the amount of acid-producing parietal cells are reduced. In addition, gastric emptying increases and intra-abdominal pressure decreases as total weight decreases. These may explain the improvement in symptoms without HH repair.

Soricelli et al. [32] published 6 patients who underwent HH repair during LSG. In 2 patients with hiatal defects larger than 5 cm, polypropylene mesh was suitable following crus repair, while crus repair was performed with 2 or 3 sutures with non-absorbable suture materials in the other 4 patients. No complications were observed during or after the operation, but HH recurrence was detected in 1 (17%) patient during long-term follow-up. In the literature, there are authors suggesting to use bio-absorbable mesh if HH repair is required during LSG, or to fix the remaining stomach to the colonic mucosa with bio-absorbable mesh, thus preventing both migration in the remaining stomach and possible volvulus [33, 34]. Occlusion of the esophagus due to imprisoned HH in the early postoperative period secondary to crus repair can be seen as a very rare complication. To the best of our knowledge, only one case was reported by Mizrahi et al. [35] in the literature. This potential complication does not change the fact that it is safe to perform HH repair if necessary during LSG. We think that conversion to Laparoscopic Roux and Y gastric bypass (LRYGB), in which the alimentary limb is fixed to the diaphragm, is the most appropriate option due to the presence of a short intra-abdominal esophagus and the tension in the sleeved stomach in patients where LSG and hiatoplasty are applied together and no success is achieved. Our biggest concern in the reoperation was how to prevent the reherniation of the stomach with a tube. While making our decision, we considered that the transition to LRYGB could provide several advantages; (1) it is an anti-reflux procedure in itself, (2) traction produced by the small intestine anatomically placed in the gastric pouch can help hold the stomach in place (3) Unlike LGS, it is a low pressure system. Also, fixing the blind loop of the alimentary limb to the diaphragm provides further fixation.

With regard to strengthening the hiatal repair with a patch, it is performed in symptomatic cases where the hiatal defect is >5 cm (detected intraoperatively) and where it is not possible to bring the cruses closer together without tension. Nocca et al. [12] and our experience it has been proven that this technique significantly reduces the recurrence rate of HH in patients with a hiatal defect >5 cm.

In cases, crural repair was performed by means of two or three interrupted non-absorbable stitches (**Figures 1-3**), while in the two cases with a HH > 5 cm, a U shaped polypropylene mesh was superimposed to aid crural closure.

4. Conclusions

When hiatal hernias are seen preoperatively or intraoperatively for bariatric surgery, surgical correction should ideally be made with mesh reinforcement to prevent further clinical progression. Prosthetic reinforcement of the hiatal closure should be performed in selected cases where an increased risk of HH recurrence exists. To evaluate the effectiveness of this procedure and as well as the feasibility and safety of prosthetic hiatal closure, further series with larger numbers of patients and longer follow-up are needed.

Conflict of interest

The authors declare no conflict of interest.

Author details

Seyfi Emir[1], Hasan Erdem[2], Mehmet Gençtürk[2], Muhammed Said Dalkılıç[2], Abdullah Şişik[2] and Selim Sözen[3]*

1 Department of General Surgery, Reyap Çorlu Hospital, Tekirdağ, Turkey

2 Department of General Surgery, Istanbul Obesity Surgery (IOC), Kurtköy Ersoy Hospital, Istanbul, Turkey

3 Department of General Surgery, Sözen Surgery Clinic, Istanbul, Turkey

*Address all correspondence to: selimsozen63@yahoo.com

IntechOpen

© 2022 The Author(s). Licensee IntechOpen. This chapter is distributed under the terms of the Creative Commons Attribution License (http://creativecommons.org/licenses/by/3.0), which permits unrestricted use, distribution, and reproduction in any medium, provided the original work is properly cited.

References

[1] Nocon M, Labenz J, Willich SN. Lifestyle factors and symptoms of gastro-oesophageal reflux: A population-based study. Alimentary Pharmacology & Therapeutics. 2006;**23**:169-174

[2] Kang JH, Le QA. Effectiveness of bariatric surgical procedures. A systematic review and network meta-analysis of randomized controlled trials. Medicine. 2017;**96**:e8632

[3] Stenard F, Iannelli A. Laparoscopic sleeve gastrectomy and gastroesophageal reflux. World Journal of Gastroenterology. 2015;**21**:10348-10357

[4] Chang VW, Langa KM, Weir D, Iwashyna TJ. The obesity paradox and incident cardiovascular disease: A population-based study. PLoS One. 2017;**12**:e0188636

[5] Ng M, Fleming T, Robinson M, Thomson B, Graetz N, Margono C. Global, regional and national prevalence of overweight and obesity in children and adults 1980-2013: A systematic analysis. Lancet. 2014;**384**:766-781

[6] Kasotakis G, Mittal SK, Sudan R. Combined treatment of symptomatic massive paraesophageal hernia in the morbidly obese. JSLS. 2011;**15**:188-192

[7] Wilson LJ, Ma W, Hirschowitz BI. Association of obesity with hiatal hernia and esophagitis. The American Journal of Gastroenterology. 1999;**94**:2840-2844

[8] Dutta SK, Arora M, Kireet A, Bashandy H, Gandsas A. Upper gastrointestinal symptoms and associated disorders in morbidly obese patients: A prospective study. Digestive Diseases and Sciences. 2009;**54**:1243-1246

[9] Schneider JH, Küper M, Königsrainer A, Brücher B. Transient lower esophageal sphincter relaxation in morbid obesity. Obesity Surgery. 2009;**19**:595-600

[10] Morgenthal CB, Lin E, Shane MD, Hunter JG, Smith CD. Who will fail laparoscopic Nissen fundoplication? Preoperative prediction of long-term outcomes. Surgical Endoscopy. 2007;**21**(11):1978-1984

[11] Gulkarov I, Wetterau M, Ren CJ, Fielding GA. Hiatal hernia repair at the initial laparoscopic adjustable gastric band operation reduces the need for reoperation. Surgical Endoscopy. 2008;**22**(4):1035-1041

[12] Nocca D, Krawczykowsky D, Bomans B, Noel P, Picot MC, Blanc PM, et al. A prospective multicenter study of 163 sleeve gastrectomies: Results at 1 and 2 years. Obesity Surgery. 2008;**18**(5):560-565

[13] Prachand VN, Alverdy JC. Gastroesophageal reflux disease and severe obesity: Fundoplication or bariatric surgery? World Journal of Gastroenterology. 2010;**16**:3757-3761

[14] Yang P, Chen B, Xiang S, Lin XF, Luo F, Li W. Long-term outcomes of laparoscopic sleeve gastrectomy versus rouxen- Y gastric bypass for morbid obesity: Results from a metaanalysis of randomized controlled trials. Surgery for Obesity and Related Diseases. 2019;**15**:546-555

[15] Kohn GP, Price RR, DeMeester SR, Zehetner J, Muensterer OJ, Awad Z, et al. Guidelines for the management of hiatal hernia. Surgical Endoscopy. 2013;**27**:4409-4428

[16] Baumann T, Grueneberger J, Pache G, Kuesters S, Marjanovic G, Kulemann B, et al. Three-dimensional stomach analysis with computed tomography after laparoscopic sleeve gastrectomy: Sleeve dilation and thoracic migration. Surgical Endoscopy. 2011;**25**:2323-2329

[17] Saber AA, Shoar S, Khoursheed M. Intra-thoracic sleeve migration (ITSM): An underreported phenomenon after laparoscopic sleeve gastrectomy. Obesity Surgery. 2017;**27**:1917-1923

[18] Daes J, Jimenez M, Said N, Daza J, Dennis R. Laparoscopic sleeve gastrectomy: Symptoms of gastroesophageal reflux can be reduced by changes in surgical technique. Obesity Surgery. 2012;**22**:1874-1879

[19] Mahawar K, Carr W, Jennings N, Balupuri S, Small P. Simultaneous sleeve gastrectomy and hiatus hernia repair: A systematic review. Obesity Surgery. 2015;**25**:159-166

[20] Rebecchi F, Allaix ME, Patti MG, Schlottmann F, Morino M. Gastroesophageal reflux disease and morbid obesity: To sleeve or not to sleeve? World Journal of Gastroenterology. 2017;**23**:2269-2275

[21] Rosenthal RJ, Diaz AA, Arvidsson D, et al. International sleeve gastrectomy expert panel. International sleeve gastrectomy expert panel consensus statement: Best practice guidelines based on experience of >12,000 cases. Surgery for Obesity and Related Diseases. 2012;**8**:8-19

[22] Gibson SC, Le Page PA, Taylor CJ. Laparoscopic sleeve gastrectomy: Review of 500 cases in single surgeon Australian practice. ANZ Journal of Surgery. 2015;**85**:673-677

[23] Che F, Nguyen B, Cohen A, Nguyen NT. Prevalence of hiatal hernia in the morbidly obese. Surgery for Obesity and Related Diseases. 2014;**9**(6):920-924

[24] Pham DV, Protyniak B, Binenbaum SJ, Squillaro A, Borao FJ. Simultaneous laparoscopic paraesophageal hernia repair and sleeve gastrectomy in the morbidly obese. Surgery for Obesity and Related Diseases. 2014;**10**(2):257-261

[25] Jossart GH. Routine hiatal hernia repair to prevent GERD after sleeve gastrectomy. Bariatric Times. 2011; **8**(Suppl. 5):15-16

[26] Korwar V, Peters M, Adjepong S, Sigurdsson A. Laparoscopic hiatus hernia repair and simultaneous sleeve gastrectomy: A novel approach in the treatment of gastroesophageal reflux disease associated with morbid obesity. Journal of Laparoscopic Advance Surgery Technology. 2009;**19**:761-763

[27] Clapp B. Prosthetic bioabsorbable mesh for hiatal hernia repair during sleeve gastrectomy. JSLS. 2013;**17**:641-644

[28] Huddy JR, Sr M, Ni MA, et al. Laparoscopic repair of hiatus hernia: Does mesh type influence outcome? A meta-analysis and European survey study. Surgical Endoscopy. 2016;**30**(12):5209-5221

[29] Snyder B, Wilson E, Wilson T, Mehta S, Bajwa K, Klein C. A randomized trial comparing reflux symptoms in sleeve gastrectomy patients with or without hiatal hernia repair. Surgery for Obesity and Related Diseases. 2016;**12**(9):1681-1688

[30] Santonicola A, Angrisani L, Cutolo P, Formisano G, Iovino P. The effect of laparoscopic sleeve gastrectomy with or without hiatal hernia repair on

gastroesophageal reflux disease in obese patients. Surgery for Obesity and Related Diseases. Mar-Apr 2014;**10**(2):250-255

[31] Dakour Aridi HN, Tamim H, Mailhac A, Safadi BY. Concomitant hiatal hernia repair with laparoscopic sleeve gastrectomy is safe: Analysis of the ACS-NSQIP database. Surgery for Obesity and Related Diseases. Mar 2017;**13**(3):379-384

[32] Soricelli E, Casella G, Rizzello M, Calì B, Alessandri G, Basso N. Initial experience with laparoscopic crural closure in the management of hiatal hernia in obese patients undergoing sleeve gastrectomy. Obesity Surgery. 2010;**20**:1149-1153

[33] Levine MS, Carucci LR. Imaging of bariatric surgery: Normal anatomy and postoperative complications. Radiology. 2014;**270**:327-341

[34] de Godoy EP, Coelho D. Gastric sleeve fixation strategy in laparoscopic vertical sleeve gastrectomy. Arquivos Brasileiros de Cirurgia Digestiva. 2013;**26**(Suppl. 1):79-82

[35] Mizrahi I, Tabak A, Grinbaum R, Beglaibter N, Eid A, Simanovsky N, et al. The utility of routine postoperative upper gastrointestinal swallow studies following laparoscopic sleeve gastrectomy. Obesity Surgery. 2014;**24**:1415-1419